"Hardhitting, yet tender ... A testimony to the great courage and growth that this woman has achieved ... It is a rich, life-changing experience to read this book."

—*NEW THOUGHT*

This powerful book is the unforgettable account of how a mother and son's love for each other helped them tap their inner strength in the face of an unspeakable tragedy. Here is an enduring testament to the healing power of compassion, forgiveness and love in the face of catastrophic illness . . . and a supportive and inspiring sourcebook that provides:

- Practical strategies for maintaining a physically and psychologically restorative environment, whether in the home or within a health care institution

- Invaluable guidance on alternative treatments, from homeopathic healing aids to morale-strengthening attitudinal therapies

- Psychological self-help techniques for overcoming fear and banishing negativity—for AIDS patients as well as their caregivers

- A guide to the national support groups, clinics, and workshops which, in conjunction with effective medical care, promote emotional and physical well-being

"Extraordinary ... A source of strength and inspiration."

—LOUISE TATE, DIRECTOR,
HOSPICE IN THE HOME

BETTYCLARE MOFFATT has written numerous books. She has done counseling and public speaking in the field of holistic healing, and now works extensively with various AIDS help groups.

WHEN SOMEONE
YOU LOVE HAS AIDS

A Book of Hope for Family and Friends

BettyClare Moffatt

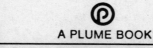

A PLUME BOOK

NAL PENGUIN INC.

NEW YORK AND SCARBOROUGH, ONTARIO

PUBLISHER'S NOTE

The ideas, procedures, and suggestions contained in this book are not intended
as a substitute for consulting with your physician. All matters regarding your health
require medical supervision.

Copyright © 1986 by BettyClare Moffatt

All rights reserved

Published by arrangement with the author.

 PLUME TRADEMARK REG. U.S. PAT. OFF. AND FOREIGN COUNTRIES
REGISTERED TRADEMARK—MARCA REGISTRADA
HECHO EN CHICAGO, U.S.A.

SIGNET, SIGNET CLASSIC, MENTOR, ONYX, PLUME, MERIDIAN
and NAL BOOKS are published *in the United States*
by NAL PENGUIN INC., 1633 Broadway, New York, New York 10019,
in Canada by The New American Library of Canada Limited,
81 Mack Avenue, Scarborough, Ontario M1L 1M8

Library of Congress Cataloging-in-Publication Data:

Moffatt, BettyClare
  When someone you love has aids.

  1. AIDS (Disease)—Popular works. 2. AIDS (Disease)—
Patients—Family relationships. 3. AIDS (Disease)—
Religious aspects. I. Title.
[RC607.A26M64 1987]   248.8′6   86-32246
ISBN 0-452-25945-2

Designed by Fritz Metsch

First Plume Printing, April, 1987

  3 4 5 6 7 8 9 10

PRINTED IN THE UNITED STATES OF AMERICA

For Michael,
In Love and Acceptance

Contents

Acknowledgments

The people who have touched my life during the year of writing this book are too numerous to mention. The personal interviews, the questionnaires, the support groups; all helped to make this book a living reality.

The entire staff of the "Love Your Self—Heal Your Body" Center were helpful, with a special acknowledgment to Gisela Miller.

I also want to thank James Baker and Jeffrey Boggs of the "Expect a Miracle" seminars; the AIDS Project, L.A.,; David Kessler of Progressive Nursing Services; and Gerald Jampolsky, M.D., for permission to quote from their fine material.

A special thank-you to Robert N. Brooks, M.D., for his insightful contribution on the medical aspects of AIDS, and his fine work with the "Being Well—Being Gay"—AIDS seminars.

The members of my family were extremely supportive, and I want to acknowledge my mother, Helen Cook, for her contribution to the book and to my life.

Finally, a special thanks to three people who helped to make this book a reality: Michael Welsch, Robert Welsch, and Steve Parrish. You know how much I love you!

INTRODUCTION

This is a book of hope. For every person who has contracted AIDS (Acquired Immune Deficiency Syndrome) it is estimated that this devastating illness will affect the lives of from five to twenty-five others, sometimes many more, as the person-patient reaches out to family, friends, lovers, coworkers, and health professionals. Like the proverbial stone dropped into a still pool, the reverberations spread ever outward, changing the lives of everyone connected, by even the slightest thread, to the person-patient with the (seemingly) incurable disease. Although AIDS is *not* a homosexual disease (Haitians are said to contract it primarily through heterosexual contact, and hemophiliacs and some children have contracted it through nonsexual means), the fact that in the United States the gay male population has been the most severely affected has made the public reaction to the problem incredibly difficult.

AIDS affects everyone it touches. It forces us to examine and work through our deepest feelings and our most hidden fears. It requires us to look at how we feel about sex, about homosexuality, about a "loathsome" plaguelike disease. It makes us examine our values, our religious convictions, our liberal or rigid stand concerning social mores. It forces those of us who are in contact with an AIDS patient to reexamine our commitments toward touching and loving and caring for a person with AIDS. Do we, especially the parents of persons with AIDS, deny our love to our children? Do we, because of social conditioning and scare tactics in the media, consign that person to the garbage pail (hurry up and die because I can't stand this anymore)? Do we scold, lecture, reject? Do we treat the child we love as a leper, as do many of his friends and colleagues, and certainly the great mass of society we come in contact with, through job-related discrimination and even the refusal of many doctors and dentists to treat the AIDS person?

Or do we use this time, the precious time, to reach out in hope and love? Do we confront our anger, frustration, fear, grief, and guilt and go forward, nurturing ourselves as we heal our families, as we reach out through whatever healing methods are available, to help our loved one who has AIDS to heal himself?

Do we reexamine our consciences and our commitment as the fight for life—*life*—continues?

Some AIDS patients live for six months, others for a year, some for two; some, for all we know of remission at this time, choose to live as long as they like. William Calderon, of San Francisco, beat the odds for over seven years. He chose to be an inspiration to others, a beacon of hope that reminds us that "Nothing is impossible." Others have chosen to use whatever time they have to increase the quality of their lives, to clear up relationships, so that each moment of life is precious and well lived.

I am a mother of a son, Michael, who had AIDS. At the time this book was first written, Michael was both living and learning through his illness. I chose to help him in his quest for life and, through this book, to present a way of being in the world, a way of loving in the world, that can, I sincerely believe, help other mothers, other fathers, all those with a family structure; indeed, all who are part of the matrix that makes up connections around the AIDS person.

This book is a journey through life and death, through hope and health. The practical aspects of living with an AIDS person are here. The statistics (numbers on a page that change daily) are here. And the tools for living in a loving way are here.

When I become terrified at the thought of loss, of death, I often use the phrase "fear forward" as a talisman to light me through the dark. It is a way of telling myself that I am here in this body to confront my fears and move through them, not to run away, not to dwell on the fears and stay with them or wallow in them, but to go through them and past them, like a laser beam of light that takes the unbearable feelings in me and transforms them into action.

This book is my "fear forward" book. May the ideas and suggestions bring hope, help, and healing into your life, as they have for me.

"I am not the victim of the world I see."
—A COURSE IN MIRACLES

=1= "MOTHER, I HAVE AIDS."

My son Michael called me from San Francisco in May of 1985.

"Mother," he said, his voice breaking. "I have something to tell you."

"How are you, darling?"

Thank you, God, that Michael is calling me, when he has been so distant, so closed-in, since he ran away from home at age fifteen, twelve years earlier. The last time I had seen him was almost a year before, when my grandson, Zachary, had died and Michael had come back to Texas for the funeral. There, at a time of great sadness for all of us, I had been able to get through to Michael, to really connect with him as I had not been able to do through years of phone calls and letters and occasional visits to San Francisco.

Michael had been ill a lot lately. He hadn't wanted me to be there for him; instead he had relied on Nancy, his ex-stepmother, who lived only a block from him. He relied on her when his atopic dermatitis flared into shingles. He had relied on her when fungal meningitis struck, incapacitating him for weeks. Because Michael was always secretive,

4

the rest of the family, including me, found out about his illnesses and hospitalizations only after the fact.

"At least he has Nancy."

I often comforted myself with that thought. "At least, he is not alone."

But now that I had moved across the country to Santa Monica, I was closer, and wanted to be closer still, to this third son I loved so much.

"Mother," he said again, "are you sitting down?"

Fear came up into my throat. I waited an eternity for the fateful words to drop into my heart.

"Mother, I have AIDS."

I had already known it at a deep, visceral level, but I had refused to admit the possibility in daylight hours. The AIDS epidemic was full-blown, and Michael was a prime candidate for the disease. The facts: Michael was homosexual, with skin problems and easy infections besieging him since his teenage years. Now the recent illnesses (how many and for how long?) had combined with the hiddenness of his life, the aloneness, too, to bring on this disease. ("Michael, dear Michael, child of my heart. Let me in.")

"And, Mother," he went on, his voice resolute, "I'm going to beat it. I'm going to live."

"Of course you are, darling. I have no doubt."

I kept my voice steady. Be there for him. Be there for him at last, now when he will finally let you in, will finally let you love him, now while he is still— I cut the thought off.

"I'm here for you, Michael. I love you and I'm here for you. Now, what can we do together to beat this?"

You will live, my mind was screaming. You will live, Michael. I won't let you die. And then the other thought, the unbidden but impossible-to-ignore thought, the folk-wisdom proverb passed down to me from my Texas upbringing: It's always the mother's fault. Of course it is. It's your fault that he left home at age fifteen; it's your fault he's a homosexual. It's your fault for every illness he ever had; it's your fault that he has this hideous, life-threatening disease. It's always the mother's fault.

In the midst of reassuring Michael of my unconditional love and support, in the midst of funneling energy straight to him through the telephone, funneling hope, funneling determination, all my energies concentrated on channeling to Michael my strength and my love. Only afterward, when I said good-bye and hung up the phone and put my head down on my desk and wept for the teenager I could not keep with me, wept for the young man with a death sentence hanging over his head, only then did I abandon myself to the thought, But who will help *me?*

How selfish, how self-serving to have these thoughts of fear! For mothers should always be perfect, shouldn't they? And I had promised to be there for Michael. Yet the thoughts went on. I could not stop them. Who will hold me up, who will tell me it's all right, who will be there for me when I fall apart and when I doubt? Who will help me to live?

I called upon all the faith and strength and belief in God that had helped me through years of devastation, but it seemed, at that moment, that God was not there for me.

"Where are You, God, in all this? My God, my God, why hast thou forsaken me?"

Families are never easy to explain. The dynamics of my own family, the bonds of love and caring, and the despair when love seems *not* to work, when the nuclear family blows up again and again, positive and negative forces that play against one another; how could this ever be explained to anyone outside the family? And everyone's perception of the truth changes, like a child's kaleidoscope that forms and reforms in shifting patterns of light and color, shifting patterns that fall together and apart; like families do.

And so began a personal odyssey, a way back to *life*. For every mother, father, brother, sister, grandparent, friend, lover who has a loved one who has contracted AIDS, this is a book of hope. Not a panacea but a loving, personal, practical book of hope. The truth for you and me is this: For every person who contracts AIDS, the entire family circle carries the consequences of that person's disease with them and carries, as well, the consequences of that AIDS person's decision to live hopefully or die despairingly. For every lover and every friend, for coworkers and health professionals, the AIDS person (not victim!) stands as a mirror for all our fears about disease, about death, about pain, about loss. Each one of us is confronted daily by our own deepest fears, our own personal response to life and death, our own choices to run away or to stay and love. In this connection the AIDS person serves as a metaphor for all our deepest fears about disease and death (as well as our guilt over sex), and serves us well, in love, together with the one who confronts and triumphs over a tragic diagnosis. It is my personal belief that each person who has AIDS chooses at some point, unconsciously and consciously, to live or to die—chooses at some point the length of time and the quality of that time; to be, or not to be, in this world.

We who feel so helpless, so angry at the "trick" that fate has played on the AIDS person (and by implication on us) can choose ourselves *how* we love in the face of death; we choose how we will play (at whatever level of commitment) out our own choices, how we will *live* alongside the person who has contracted AIDS.

"I am not a victim" is the first step back from death into life for the AIDS person. And "You are not a victim" was the first step forward for me, a daily, hourly reminder to myself as I confronted my feelings when told of Michael's illness.

And you and you and you and you, the mother, the father, the sister, the brother, the lover, the friend, the child—all those who come into the orbit of the AIDS person:

You are not a victim! This I say to you out of the deepest struggle within my own heart and mind and body and spirit.

We are here to learn our own lessons of living and loving. We are here *only* to learn how to love. Ultimately the choice for the duration and quality of life depends on the AIDS person himself, but we can help.

As we are all altered, in some degree, by each contact we make with each individual of the human race, we can, along with the AIDS person, choose that the contact be one of love, unconditional love, or one of fear. Choosing fear, we are bound then by every exterior evidence that adds to our mounting hysteria. We are then as "helpless" as the AIDS person. We are two "victims," two who "lose," two who are annihilated by something mysterious "out there."

Those of us who choose love, who choose life in all its magnificence, in spite of the agony, are strengthened, are transformed, are *healed*. The healing and the love come from within and are as valid a response as that of fear.

Those we love who have AIDS make their own choices daily. We can honor their choices, as we honor and cherish our relationship with them.

Those who have AIDS and those of us within and around the design of their lives have a unique opportunity to accelerate our own growth, our own capacity for love.

Could it be, perhaps, that on one level the AIDS person has "chosen" what he or she wishes to learn on the planet Earth in this lifetime, in an accelerated, speeded-up fashion?

In facing the threat of death courageously, we *can* and *must* move *through* all the stages of fear to the powerful acceptance of love, and to "living out" in our daily lives the ramifications of that power until we are, indeed, practicing unconditional love.

"There is no cruelty in God
and none in me."
—A COURSE IN MIRACLES

=2= UNDERSTANDING WORKS BOTH WAYS

When we face the stages of grief that accompany the realization of loss or the fear of loss when someone we love has AIDS, we must be prepared to deal with shockwaves of disbelief, anger, guilt, fear, sadness, frustration, and a host of any and all emotions that anyone could possibly feel. Yet our feelings are as valid as the feelings of the AIDS person.

It is vitally important, if communication and love are to take place, that the AIDS person put himself into the mind and heart of the person he is telling his story to and experience (like the proverbial man who walked a mile in someone else's moccasins), what it feels like to *be* that parent faced with this immense fear-producing, seemingly unsolvable threat to life.

Just as the homosexual person wishes so much that his parents and the entire "straight" community understand him, so it is not unreasonable for him to allow himself to understand *them*. This is a point too often overlooked by the homosexual community.

Understanding and acceptance come from where we are inside and then flow outward into the world. If you, as a

homosexual, are coming from a place of defensiveness, frustration, fear, and covert guilt, is it any wonder that family
members may not react, at first, with unconditional love?
Acceptance works both ways.

When you reach out to share the essence of yourself
with your parents and other relatives, all who comprise the
family structure, you create a climate where meaningful
dialogue can take place. This goes far beyond Gay Pride or a
fanatical zeal to convert everyone to your own point of view.
The truth is that your parents and other family members
have a lifetime of social and moral conditioning that may
certainly preclude instant acceptance, but seldom, if ever,
preclude love. For the homosexual and/or AIDS person,
asking for acceptance, healing help, and love, it is wise to be
both realistic and empathic with where your parents are
coming from. Belief systems are deeply entrenched. It often
takes a family crisis like AIDS for barriers between families
to fall away. Asking for understanding is one thing. Asking
for approval is another. Unconditional love is not solely the
province of mothers. Unconditional love is a two-way street.

I recall a meeting I attended recently wherein homosexual men and women (none of whom had AIDS) came together with their friends, lovers, parents (usually mothers,
as mothers are far more inclined generally to reach out and
respond lovingly, more willing to change emotionally, more
willing to be the catalyst in healing family divisions).

During the course of the meeting we broke up into
several small circular groups, where on hard, straight-backed
chairs on possibly the hottest day of the year, we sat in those
"hot seats" and "rapped" with each other. All too often the
group's avowed purpose of empathy and attempts to help the
straight parent or friend to come to terms with the shocking
truth about their loved son or daughter was destroyed or
rendered ineffective by the obduracy of the gay family member.

An older woman who had just found out that her only

son was gay, and who was in tears at the very thought of such a thing happening in her life, was immobilized by her own guilt at "failing" to bring up her son alone while struggling to support them both as a single parent. She was bewildered, shocked, angry. She was literally mourning the loss of the person she thought her teenage son had been for sixteen years, while struggling to accept his orientation as other than a shameful fact to be kept hidden from her employers and friends and other family members. So it was with incredulity that I observed the insensitivity of one young man in the group, who sneered at her tears, blandly ignored her halting questions to understand, and dismissed her feelings with this glib censorious statement: "You should," he advised her, "quit that crying and be glad your son has a good place to come where he can find a lover. Why," he went on, "I'd be glad to introduce him to a sweetie pie for him right here."

Considering the feeling state of the mother, the young gay man's remarks made me flinch. In this case, the words *insensitive* and *uncaring* applied not to the mother but to the young man, supposedly enlightened, who was "trying to help her."

The evening there seemed full of anger and fear, coming mostly from the very people who professed to help. It's as if the negatives associated with our society, including our own cultural bias, our fear and rage at someone behaving differently from us, were twisted in such a way that those of us who came to help heal and be healed were rather the recipients of various diatribes. Our own feelings were not honored. Our struggle was seen as inconsequential. Our willingness to understand and love and accept the gay person in our family was merely a fortuitous way for us to be attacked for our own long, deeply held, and entrenched belief systems.

I had come as a counselor and a mother. I left feeling

drained, depleted, and depressed at the apparent inability of the two worlds to connect and communicate, much less understand and forgive differences.

Another mother left when I did. She had been in a group whose chief purpose, it seemed to her, was for a young gay woman to rail against her employers when she was asked to remove certain sexual appurtances from her desk, as well as sexual magazines they objected to in the workplace.

"I was just trying to educate them," she explained. "I told them just what I thought of them and what they could do with the material in graphic detail."

The mother was crying as she told this, and I reached out to hug her as she went on, "I have a daughter who is gay. And I came here for help. I want to understand. But all of this is so distasteful to me. Does it get any better?" she wondered aloud. "Do I lay aside all my upbringing, my sense of what is right or wrong, all the moral and social dos and don'ts? Do I admit, as the people in the group seemed to insist on, that I have been wrong all these years, that I have been ignorant, uninformed, prejudiced? It's one thing for people to have Gay Pride," she went on, "but what about my *own* pride? What about *my* feelings? Does there have to be a wrong or right about heterosexuality and homosexuality? Can't there be understanding on both sides?"

Another mother (there are a lot of us out there) told me, "I feel like a stranger in a strange land. I'm willing to learn and accept what my son is all about. I'm willing to let him go and accept whomever and however he loves. But why," she asked, "can't my son behave in a loving manner toward me? He shoves unpalatable truths at me and demands instant understanding and unconditional love. He expects me to accept certain areas of his life that I *do* feel uneasy about. He expects me to condone his "cruising" and his flamboyant behavior, yet he withholds his love from me. 'I'll forgive you, Mother,' he says, magnanimously, 'for not understanding me in the past. I'll forgive you, Mother, for not being the perfect mother I expected and demanded. I forgive you, Mother.' For what?" she went on rhetorically, saddened and bewildered rather than angry. "All of us do the best we can with who we are. Why should I be punished and made to feel guilty when I reach out to my son, when I do not punish him or try to make him feel guilty? Love is *not* one-sided. Understanding, compassion, forgiveness are not one-sided. I am willing to change my ideas and expectations of what my son 'should' be. Why, then, can't he do the same for me? In his eyes I was not the mother I 'should' have been. Well, I did a damn good job under incredible circumstances, and I deserve more!"

We cannot ask people to be what they are not. Just as we cannot ask our sons or daughters to be like us, just as adulthood entails autonomy and responsibility for one's choices, just so are we entitled to be who we are, mother, father, grandparent, aunt, uncle, child, friend. Separateness polarizes. Acceptance unites. The fear of the gay community toward the straight community is as pervasive and cruel as the fear of the straight community toward the gay community. Neither has all the answers. Neither is morally superior to the other.

All of this may sound as if the only people to contract AIDS are gay men. This is simply not true! However, since the majority of AIDS cases at this time have as their common denominator the young gay male homosexuals, it is certainly relevant to acknowledge the fear and anger that are components of any and all family mourning. This fear and anger are escalated for many of us upon learning that our sons are both homosexual and dying. (Or so the doctors say at this point.)

Allow us time to mourn. This is the message for all those reading this book. Whether you are gay or straight, whether you are a family member, lover or friend, whether you are a coworker or helping professional, allow those of us who have just learned the truth about our loved one's illness to go through our own grief.

In *Living With Loss*, Drs. Ronald W. Ramsey and Rene Noorbergen discuss the stages that most people go through when faced with loss, whether it be that of death, divorce, surgery, or other major life crises. Subtitled *A Dramatic Breakthrough in Grief Therapy*, the book is valuable for its insistence on the grieving persons coming to terms with the loss by *confronting* their emotions and moving through these emotions by completely experiencing them. They mention the five stages of grief that most people go through when faced with a life crisis of the first magnitude: initial shock, intense sadness, withdrawal from the environment, protest of the loss, a gradual resolution of the loss. By experiencing these stages (which cannot be hurried), the person involved in the life crisis can then, and only then, go on to the rest of his/her life, moving on to acceptance and then action.

It is my personal experience that learning of the AIDS diagnosis, combined with the disclosure of the AIDS person's life-style, compounded by the media's insistence on scaring the entire population of the Western world with its coverage of this "loathsome, incurable, plaguelike disease" leads the parent into a black hole of anger, fear, and helplessness, including the five stages of grief so succinctly covered in *Living With Loss*.

For the mother of an AIDS person a pervasive sense of guilt (false guilt, but try to tell any one of us that at the time) overlays the depression and sense of helplessness, the it's-no-use feelings. This comes at the time in which we are asked to understand, accept, love, and often physically care for the AIDS person. This comes at a time when we are feeling most useless, most impotent, less able to marshal our forces and force ourselves to smile with that stiff upper lip. When we are most vulnerable, we are asked to be strong. When we are most angry, we are expected to give unconditional love. When we are most frightened, we struggle to trust. When we feel we can't go on, we are asked to go forward with inward calm.

I recall one mother breaking down in front of me.

"I am so angry," she admitted. "I'm angry at everyone and everything. I'm angry at my son for getting this disease. I'm angry at his life-style. I'm angry at my husband for not understanding our son. I'm angry at the doctors for their fatal diagnosis. I'm angry at the other family members who think I should hide the truth about my son's illness. I'm angry at the whole damn world for not understanding what this family is going through; and I'm especially angry at myself, for *having* this anger!"

For another young man whose brother contracted AIDS and later died, his entire Midwestern family felt only shame at the nature of the illness. They bought into the "what-will-people-think?" syndrome (a result of their own upbringing, combined with current media hysteria and their fundamentalist views). They buried their son as hastily and privately as possible, with a false death certificate and a disguised obituary so no one would know of his "perversion."

The dead man's brother was anguished.

"I will mourn my brother openly," he decided, but he found that he had to leave his parents' community in order to do so, that the climate of understanding and support he sought while he went through his stages of grief was denied him.

It is imperative that each of us experience our total feelings, not just those acceptable to us or to the people around us, in order to come to terms with this illness of our loved one. More than coming to terms, we must not be denied our grief. We must not deny ourselves, nor allow others to deny us, our honest feelings, *all of them,* no matter how unacceptable they may be to us at the time.

Even the AIDS person is sometimes guilty of neither understanding, nor accepting what his parents are going through. Michael's stepmother advised him, "Let me have my grief. Let me have my time of mourning. And let your mother and your father have their feelings, *all* their feelings. Out of that will come their strength and their acceptance." She said this after she, respecting Michael's wish that no one else know of his illness, had witnessed two weeks in which he almost died from fungal meningitis, two weeks in which he struggled to stay alive under impossible odds. Sometime during that hospital stay she was able to come to terms with her own grief and fear. And yet she, too, had miles to go before her feelings steadied into strength and acceptance. *Then* she was able to reach out and help other family members when confronted with their initial shock of Michael's illness.

It has been said that mourning (including anger, fear, and sadness) cannot be rushed; that a death, for example, can take at least two years for all the grief to be worked through, and often much longer than that when the griever denies or conceals his or her feelings.

In my own experience I have found that when I feel my feelings most deeply, no matter how devastating and immobilizing they seem at the time, I am then able to go on in a stronger, lighter manner, able to operate with a sense of safety in a universe that all my fears cannot destroy. This has not been easy for me to learn. In fact, I am still learning this most valuable lesson. *You get through by going through.*

"In order to solve anything you have to go past the point of pain." This incredible insight came to me in a meditation training seminar many years ago, in which I was reliving and reexperiencing the pain of my children leaving home. I remember the sensation in back of my eyes as mirrors seemingly shattered into a thousand fragments along with all my pictures of my past, the grief and sense of loss that had been with me for so long. They then reformed and coalesced into a sensation in the center of my chest that was like no other pain that I can remember. It was a pain so devastating that tears rained down the corners of my closed eyes while I struggled within to breathe past the pain. It was like throwing myself against locked, armored steel doors.

It was then that the words came: "In order to solve anything, you have to go past the pain." I decided then to breathe into the pain, to dive into it, to become one with the steel door that, gradually opening to my breath, became a black hole. "In order to solve anything, you've got to get past the pain." I repeated the words again and again as a litany while I let go into the desolation of total, indescribable loss. And at the end was light. *Light!*

I remember the words and the sensation whenever I find myself struggling with people and events I cannot change, whenever I find myself in despair over what looks like death, instead of life. *You get through by going through.* Avoiding your own feelings when your child has AIDS does no good. The feelings are still there. They are *your* feelings, they are *your* pain, they are *you!* Choosing life—*life*—daily, instead of choosing death, means that you also choose to confront those fears, those abysses of anger, guilt, frustration, sadness, *all* of those feelings. Then and only then can you come through. Then and only then can you come out the other side of pain, no matter what the world outside may look like at the moment.

Then choose life! In the midst of death choose life, for a whole person is darkness as well as light, sadness as well as joy.

I have learned more in the last two years about *experiencing* the principles so easily mouthed by many. It is one thing to believe in basic universal truths; it is quite

another to take what you have learned and put it into practice. One of the areas in which I work with parents and
friends of people who have AIDS is a Monday night study
group called A Course in Miracles. It has been invaluable to
me, to Michael, and to my youngest son, Robert, as a focal
point for understanding and healing relationships. Through
this group, as well as through other support groups and
therapeutic techniques offered elsewhere in this book, I am
continually healing myself and, from that place of certainty,
reaching out to write this book.

   This course teaches us that everything is either love or
fear, and that we choose in each moment to experience one
or the other of these two states. At the same time it is my
feeling that we must go through a veil of illusion and a time
of confusion, not by ignoring our feeling states but by going
through them to the other side, which is always love and
inner peace. When we "fear forward," by going past the
point of pain and totally trusting in the light, then we are
healed, then we are made whole, then we experience acceptance, then we go on.

"I can escape from the world I see
by giving up attack thoughts."

—A COURSE IN MIRACLES

3

AIDING THE AIDS PERSON

Aiding the Parents and Friends
of the AIDS Person

Families are not easily mended. Everyone whom I have met who has AIDS or has a family member with AIDS has stories to tell of guilt, loneliness, and alienation.

Some philosopher once said that no one has a happy childhood, or at least admits to one. What I have found, in my own experience with Michael, is that on a spiritual level the AIDS person chooses (quite unconsciously) to manifest the disease known as AIDS from a deep, hidden lack of self-esteem, compounded by sexual guilt and feelings of worthlessness.

This does not condemn or condone the AIDS person. It is simply a metaphysical observation corroborated by Louise Hay, whose pioneering work with AIDS patients has helped many AIDS persons to come to terms with their feelings, *and from that point onward* make new choices about themselves and the people in their lives.

Again and again I hear stories from AIDS persons in which they *initially* blame their parents, their partners, the world, society, God (especially God!) for the disease. While this is a human reaction, it does not serve the AIDS person or his family to blame anyone or anything—past, present, or future—for what happened. Instead, what those of us who reach out to AIDS persons have seen is that the healing begins when the blaming ends.

Part of the healing happens when the AIDS person (*and everyone in his family!*) begins to take *total* responsibility for the disease "happening" to the AIDS person, and through him, outward to his family.

It goes something like this: "Because I love you, I am here for you. Therefore this is a unique opportunity for both of us to clear up any unfinished business from the past. If there are things you need to tell me from your perceptions of your childhood, fine. If there are feelings to share that lead both of us toward understanding, good. If, on the other hand, you want to work out your feelings privately or with the aid of a trusted therapist or support group, that is fine too.

"However"—and this is a big one—"the purpose of sharing our feelings is not to punish or to blame. The purpose of sharing our feelings is just that—to share who I am with who you are, to share past pains only to eradicate them, to share past loving thoughts and feelings as well."

The past itself is over.

What is important are the conclusions one has about events of the past. There are many techniques to discover these conclusions. One potent and intense therapeutic technique, "rebirthing" (conscious connected breathing while working with a trained facilitator in order to discover and release childhood conclusions that have led to current states of being and behaving in the world), is one way to get back to root causes that may very well have originated at the moment of birth. At that time the person may have concluded, "Life hurts. No one loves me. I'm all alone. I'm helpless. I'm weak. I'm not good enough."

While all of us may at times have these feelings, the

AIDS person, in his detectivelike zeal to unearth the causes behind his current place in space and time, cannot *afford* to conclude, "Aha! My father or mother did not love me enough at birth. It's all their fault I'm the way I am now." Again the past is irrelevant. Only the *conclusions* drawn from the past need to be changed.

As a parent, I am often filled with guilt feelings about all the "mistakes" I made with my children. I can tell myself that I was only seventeen when my first son was born, and certainly, at that point, not equipped with perfect, wise, loving, mothering skills, but what I really remember about my later mothering experiences is holding each of my four sons in my arms and telling each one, "I love you, and I'm going to take care of you the best I can."

When a person has AIDS, the whole family gets a miraculous second chance to heal all the human mistakes that may have led all of them to this point in time.

A Course in Miracles states: "When I am healed, I am not healed alone."

How incredible it is, then, to have a grown son turn to you and say, "Mother, you're not at all the way I have been thinking about you all these years. Mother, I love you and I want you in my life."

If it is indeed true that every action creates an equal reaction, then love and acceptance will have to flower and flow from both ends of the spectrum. The adult son or daughter with AIDS is just as capable of making his or her parents feel guilty as the parent is capable of responding in kind.

Give us time to learn who you are. Give us time to work through our own feelings about what this disease means to us. Give us time to reflect, to absorb, to assimilate, to be there for you in an emergency. And if we do not respond perfectly, if first or second overtures are met inappropriately (as the therapists say), then give us time to work through our fears, our hostility, our own (often false and misapplied) guilt. Give us time to find out who we are when tragedy hits. Allow us to be human. Allow us to rage and mourn, as we allow you the same privilege.

"I did not make you sick," explained one mother to her son. "You are not a victim of the past. So don't victimize me!"

AIDS can be an intense, incredible journey through the stages of life and death when the patient stops being a victim of his past and takes full and total responsibility for his present situation and, through that total commitment, creates the future he wants.

AIDS can be the catalyst that brings a family together, but again, every family member is responsible for his or her own actions or feelings. We can't turn on the symphony orchestra and have the weeping parents say at once, "No matter what, I am here for you," although in some cases, that is what actually happens. We also can't expect the AIDS person to say, "Gee, Ma (or Pa), I'm so sorry I upset you by contracting this loathsome disease. I promise I'll never do it again." Both are unrealistic absurdities.

And in the midst of all the human feelings, in the midst of all the negatives, one picture stands out in my mind. At a recent positive-support meeting that did deal specifically and lovingly with the reactions of parents and coworkers to those who have AIDS, a young man with ARC (AIDS-related complex) cried as he told how his parents refused to speak to him when he told them of his disease. This man is a middle-aged successful writer whose world had crumbled. He had lost his job, his lover, and his parents' support when he "came out" with the story of his illness and his own fears. During the course of that evening a woman whose son had AIDS embraced him, held him to her heart in love and acceptance.

"I'm here for you," she whispered. "Give them [your parents] time. I know they love you."

But the healing of family members is not accomplished overnight, and family members are not the only ones who need to learn new ways of dealing with the AIDS person. While it is obviously beyond the scope of this book to educate the entire general public, still prevailing attitudes can and must be changed on every level in order for the AIDS person to make choices about his own healing. The following are some pervasive attitudes that hinder the AIDS person *and* family members from finding the help they so desperately need at this time of crisis.

The "Make Your Will, It's All Over but the Shouting" Syndrome

Health professionals are usually the ones most guilty of buying into the idea that the AIDS person is going to die— and fast! In the name of "telling the truth" and "biting the bullet," they diagnose and give the death sentence in the same breath. Psychiatrists and social workers are just as guilty as the medical doctors. Again and again, people with AIDS who seem to be healing (the doctors call it remission, but life by any other name can smell as sweet), are told that their lives are over.

William Calderon, the remarkable AIDS person who had been free of AIDS symptoms for over seven years, told the story of meeting the hospital psychiatrist in the elevator one day. Over a year earlier the psychiatrist had told Calderon, step by step, how he would die. The doctor, on seeing Calderon alive and well, blurted out, "What are you doing here? You're supposed to be dead."

Granted, one must know the facts, which at this point

go something like this: "You have contracted a disease called AIDS. Here are possible treatments to arrest the disease. There are also possible alternatives." Even, "Here are recent medical advances through research that are on the horizon and can offer you hope." Or, "Here are support groups and positive therapists who can help you explore your feelings and take responsibility for your life." All of the above are hopeful, life-enhancing possibilities for the AIDS person. To say instead, "Prepare to die. There is no hope," condemns the AIDS person to an authority figure's diagnosis that seems irrevocable. The swift deterioration of the AIDS person then follows the old self-fulfilling prophecy.

In my opinion it is criminally irresponsible for the health professional and/or family and friends to condemn the AIDS person to a swift and sudden death. There are choices. There are alternatives. Some of these alternatives will be explored in depth later on in this book.

It is vitally important that *you*, whoever you are and whatever your relationship with an AIDS person is, not to give up!

The Religious Know-it-all Moral Superiority Syndrome

"Take that, you sinner! You have AIDS because you are dirty, filthy, sexually depraved, a pervert, morally unfit, damned to eternal hellfire. And by implication—stop whatever you're doing and be saved by me" (one who is, of course, morally superior to you in every way). The other side of this equation (since everything is black and white, there are only two ways of looking at this), goes as follows, "Hurry up and die! And, God, be quick about it because this AIDS person offends my moral sensibilities!"

It is currently assumed that about 70% of the people

who contract AIDS are male homosexuals and/or bisexual. It is known that AIDS is spread by sexual contact or blood. Also, metaphysically speaking, people who feel guilty about their sexual practices are said to manifest whatever guilt is lodged in their bodies through the disease AIDS. Nevertheless, the 270,000 people who will have contracted AIDS by 1991 (a conservative estimate according to the Atlanta Center for Disease Control) cannot possibly all be guilty, perverted sinners. Haitians, West Africans, monkeys, elderly men of Mediterranean descent (who often manifest Kaposi's sarcoma, a cancer seen in AIDS person), hemophiliacs, others who contract the disease through blood transfusions, both heterosexuals and homosexuals, recent cases involving mothers and children, even ARC (AIDS-related complex) patients—surely all of the above cannot and must not be condemned by self-appointed moral guardians. To make sweeping moral statements about the plague of AIDS is as insane as to condemn all people who die of pneumonia or cancer as being morally unfit in some way. Condemnation serves no purpose. It helps neither the AIDS person nor the family and friends who love and care for the AIDS person. Whatever your own individual life-style or religious upbringing, whatever struggles you find within yourself when confronting your private feelings about this plague, acceptance and love will get you farther than moral condemnation any day.

If you are a caretaker or health professional, or a concerned friend or relative, keep your *human* judgments to yourself. Your hypocritical judgments serve neither you, the person with AIDS, nor the concerned family.

For those who would quote New Testament scripture, I refer them to Christ walking among the lepers (surely our AIDS persons are often treated like lepers), and also to his reminder that we should "Judge not, that ye be not judged."

Many of us who care for AIDS persons are faithful

churchgoers doing our best to live out our faith and love in devastating circumstances. The knowledge that prayer can and does work miracles does not excuse conditional, sanctimonious, judgmental prayer. To "behold the Christ in everyone" is surely more conducive to healing than "casting the first stone."

The purpose of this book is not to judge, condemn, or condone, but instead to offer avenues of hope, healing, and acceptance. It is cruel and reprehensible to treat the patient and the ones who love the AIDS person (be they homosexual or heterosexual) as if they were in fact unclean. Prayer, like love, is unconditional.

The "Squirting Whipped Cream over the Worms" Syndrome

No wonder many doctors and health professionals shun like the plague the people who blandly tell the AIDS patient, "Just think positively and you'll get well." The emphasis here is that the AIDS person is to blame for the disease (blaming yourself is not the same as taking responsibility for healing your life). The not-so-subtle message from the "positive-thinking, New Age, New Thought person" is again one of moral superiority and spiritual one-upmanship over the AIDS patient. It goes something like this: "I don't have AIDS, but you do. Therefore, since your thoughts cause disease, I am better, more enlightened, purer, smarter, and more capable of healing my life than you are." The advice given is, "Just think everything is okay, and it will be."

This approach does not take into consideration the following possibilities.

The patient may have chosen AIDS as a vehicle to transformation, but not at a conscious level. To tell a person who is frightened, angry, and in pain, fighting for his life, to merely "think the disease away" serves no one, especially not the AIDS person, who already feels guilty and despairing enough.

On the contrary, the "Squirting Whipped Cream over the Worms" syndrome leaves the worms squirming underneath to get out. The AIDS person, in the course of therapeutic self-discovery, has to look at the worms, i.e., "What in me contributes to and/or causes this disease?" and "What in me needs to be changed and uprooted so that I can heal in peace?" (Or die in peace, if that is what I so desire.)

It is not anger that kills. It is suppressed anger that kills. The AIDS person may have to "come out of the closet" with his or her anger in order for the disease to be released from the body. The AIDS person may very well have put on a happy face for years, while underneath, the resentment and rage and despair smoldered. Now it is time for soul-searching and truth-telling. Now is the time to safely express the long-buried emotions that may indeed have led to the onset of AIDS. Emotion is energy in motion. Move the energy out and the body can and will heal itself faster.

In addition to the previously mentioned therapeutic techniques such as rebirthing and AIDS support groups such as Louise Hay's (various support groups are now springing up all over the country, including my MAP group for mothers of AIDS persons), there are additional tools for combating the "Squirting Whipped Cream Over the Worms" syndrome. These include the following:

Psychological techniques that include writing long, emotional, no-holds-barred letters to those people you wish to forgive and be forgiven by (whether they are alive or not), and then burning the letters. Releasing the emotions safely through the use of boffing sticks or pounding pillows. Releasing pent-up anger through screaming in the shower, or into a pillow, or through verbalizing your anger to a trusted

therapist or friend. The key here is to let the AIDS patient
or family member express feelings. Perhaps this is the first
time he or she can tell the truth about his or her emotions.
At this point the AIDS person has nothing to lose and
everything to heal by identifying and releasing negative emotions from the body.

Meditation, visualization, and positive prayer are all
excellent approaches to healing the distress within the AIDS
person, as are spiritual study helps such as those found in
New Age study groups springing up across the nation.

Each of these approaches has but one end: to heal the
person involved by encouraging the AIDS person to take
charge of his own emotions, and by offering processes instead of platitudes. There is a vast difference between saying,
"It's your fault you have AIDS" and "Take the responsibility
for healing your life."

In my own case, experiencing *all* of the above techniques again and again and facilitating other family members, including Michael, in using these psychological and
spiritual helps to get through the initial confusion and pain,
has helped me in countless ways in my own search for
acceptance and inner peace. Loving myself enough to clear
myself continually of outmoded attitudes and overwhelming
fears has helped me get to the place where I can honestly set
down this personal and (I trust) practical journey in book
form.

My favorite quotation from Eleanor Roosevelt is taped
to the corner of my typewriter so that I can see it every day;
it says it better than I can: "In the long run, we shape our
lives, and we shape ourselves. The process never ends until
we die. And the choices we make are ultimately our own
responsibility."

4

THE MEDICAL ASPECTS
OF AIDS

In a personal journey through Michael's illness and the
world of AIDS, I have had to come to terms with certain
fearful and unpalatable facts about the AIDS virus. At the
same time that I am thinking health, the AIDS epidemic
confronts me head-on. At the same time that I am clearing
myself of old patterns of reacting to alternative life-styles, so
that I can truly serve in love and acceptance the people who
come to me concerned with the ramifications of this devastating disease, I am reminded of the statistics about AIDS. As
a traditionally brought-up mother and grandmother, it is still
very difficult for me to write of a disease that is usually
transmitted by sexual contact, a veneral disease between two
consenting adults, usually homosexual men, yet heterosexu-
ally transmittable as well.

Since this book is about confronting your deepest feelings and coming to a place of acceptance and love, I am
asking now that the reader accept the facts in this chapter
with an open mind.

The medical material presented here comes from two
sources: Robert Brooks, M.D., a Los Angeles psychiatrist

who has achieved remarkable remissions in his "Being Well—Being Gay—AIDS" practice; and intensive research done by the health professionals who contributed to a book called *Living With Aids: A Self-Care Manual,* written and distributed worldwide by the AIDS Project, Los Angeles. While statistics from the Center for Disease Control in Atlanta change daily, and while researchers around the world are working to develop a vaccine that will help the AIDS patient in his fight for life, nevertheless, at this time, it is imperative to know all we can about the disease known as AIDS, rather than relying on the media's scare tactics that emphasize the epidemic rather than all of the medical facts. To be well informed is *not* to give up and accept standard medical diagnoses. There have been too many remissions for that. The facts do exist, and since this book is intended to present material concerned with the *totality* of the mind/body/emotions/spirit connection, the body cannot be ignored.

What Is AIDS?

"Acquired Immune Deficiency Syndrome (AIDS) is the result of a defect in the immune system's ability to resist certain types of infections: those caused by viruses, fungi, parasites, and mycobacteria (tuberculosislike organisms). In addition, resistance to certain types of cancer is also diminished."
—*Living With AIDS,* The AIDS Project, Los Angeles, 1984.

What does this information mean to you and me? It means that AIDS is not a disease in itself. The mortality rate from AIDS comes from the body's inability to *resist* what is known as "opportunistic infections"—that is, the person doesn't die from AIDS. Instead, when the body's immune system is impaired, a host of illnesses can rush in. This is what is happening in the AIDS epidemic. The *Living With AIDS* description of the medical diagnosis of AIDS as affecting the immune system in ways currently under study and revision by researchers, goes on to say:

> We are limited to describing AIDS as a collection of signs, symptoms, and laboratory findings which indicate the presence of the illness. The term "acquired" is used because people with AIDS are known to have normal immune system function prior to the onset of the syndrome. The organisms listed previously (viruses, fungi, parasites, and mycobacteria) which cause infections in persons with AIDS are *commonly found in the everyday environment and do not affect individuals with normal immune system function*. [Italics mine.] When they cause infections they are called "opportunistic." Opportunistic infections are also seen in others with suppressed immune system function such as patients with leukemia or in organ transplant recipients who have had their immune system function deliberately suppressed to prevent rejection of the transplant. The difference between AIDS and leukemia, or organ transplants, is that the immune system suppression that occurs with AIDS is more severe and appears to be the result of an infectious agent (most likely a recently identified virus.)

I went to Dr. Robert Brooks, M.D., a psychiatrist whose work with AIDS patients has recently received national attention, for further medical information. The following medical paper on AIDS is reprinted here in its entirety with his permission. While statistics change daily, the basic information, while couched in medical terminology, is clear, concise, and less threatening than much of the research literature on AIDS.

The Acquired Immune Deficiency Syndrome

Since first being described, over 25,000 cases of AIDS have been reported to the Center for Disease Control. The conservative predictions are that by 1991, another 245,000 new cases will have been reported. This makes AIDS an epidemic of shocking proportions in this country, as well as world-wide.

The CDC defines AIDS as "a reliably diagnosed disease that is at least moderately indicative of an underlying cellular immunodeficiency in a person who has had no known cause of underlying cellular immunodeficiency or any other underlying reduced resistance reported to be associated with that disease."

With AIDS there is a severe problem of cellular immunity, with an absolute decrease in the number of helper T-lymphocytes. Persons with AIDS are thus rendered susceptible to a number of so called "opportunistic" infections with protozoa, fungi, certain bacteria, and viruses. Certain malignancies also occur in this group of patients; Kaposi's sarcoma is the most common, but other types have been reported.

More than 70% of AIDS patients are homosexual or bisexual men, but other groups of people also get AIDS: I.V. drug users, hemophiliacs, and others. AIDS has been reported in over 46 states, the District of Columbia, Puerto Rico, and in 21 other countries. New York, California, and Florida have reported over 75% of the U.S. cases.

Since the original description of AIDS, the most likely cause has appeared to be by infection. Recently a group of viral agents termed retroviruses has been implicated in the causation of AIDS. The human T-cell lymphotrophic virus, HTLV-III (a retrovirus), has been isolated from several patients with AIDS, antibodies thought to be pre-AIDS like. Studies have revealed antibodies to this group of viruses in over 50% of one group of persons thought to be at high risk in San Francisco.

Since not everyone with evidence of contact with this agent is developing AIDS, other factors are also working. Host resistance and nutritional factors as well as other cofactors may be responsible for the development of the disorder.

There is no single test available to diagnose AIDS. There are a number of factors which must be taken into consideration to make this diagnosis. At present, AIDS remains a clinical diagnosis. That means that the variety of symptoms, various clinical signs, and the result of certain non-specific laboratory tests must all be examined together to make the determination that a person has AIDS.

The treatment of AIDS at present is directed at management of the opportunistic infections or tumors that develop as a result of the immunodeficiency. To cure a patient would require that we could reverse the immune problem. We do not know how to do this at the present time. We are getting better at managing the infections and the tumors, and there is research in progress aimed at trying to find ways to reverse the immunodeficiency.

AIDS is transmitted by body fluids during intimate sexual contact, I.V. drug use, from a blood transfusion, or during pregnancy to a fetus.

A test for exposure to HTLV-III is now commercially available. However, this test only indicates exposure. A positive test is difficult to interpret beyond that inference. A negative test may of more value in advising a given patient. At the present time this test is advised only for screening blood prior to transfusion.

From a clinical point of view, the patient and the doctor are more concerned with the status of the immune system. This kind of information is obtained from specific immunologic tests such as T-cell subsets. In contrast to the HTLV-III antibody tests, which merely indicate past contact with the viral agent, these tests give a more precise indication of the integrity of the immune system and do not carry the social or psychological risks of being found positive for HTLV-III antibody.

Theoretically, a vaccine against HTLV-III is possible. However, the requirements of producing a vaccine that is clinically effective and safe are many, and practically speaking, the finished product is not to be expected on the market for some time. And, of course, such a vaccine will most likely be of little or no value to those persons already infected with the virus.

Since AIDS is most likely caused by an infectious agent transmitted sexually, by sharing hypodermic needles, or through blood or blood products, prevention at present rests on restricting the number and kinds of sexual contacts (especially those kinds of practices that involve ingestion or retention of infected body secretions), elimination of I.V. needle sharing, and using blood or blood products only when absolutely indicated. These recommendations will not cure the AIDS epidemic, but will certainly go a long way to reduce the spread of AIDS.

Persons at high risk for AIDS, as well as persons with AIDS, should adhere to other health practices known to enhance well-being, including adequate and appropriate exercise, adequate and balanced nutrition, sufficient rest, as well as decreasing unnecessary stress, and developing a positive emotional attitude and outlook.

I want to emphasize here that people *without* AIDS not only get opportunistic infections, but can die from them. While AIDS appears to depress the immune system from a specific virus, there are people who have severe immune deficiencies and do *not* have AIDS. My personal bout with illness is a case in point.

When I first moved from Texas to California, after going through a year of almost unbelievable stress, my body, which I had always counted on to perform magnificently no matter what (I had not had even a cold in fifteen years), collapsed totally. The diagnosis: severe immune system breakdown involving the pituitary, combined with a severe viral infection that affected the following organs: the lymph glands, the ovarian glands, the thyroid gland, the liver, the lungs, and the bronchi. In addition, a raging viral infection, involving both my ears and the above-mentioned glands, caused high fevers, night sweats, weakness, confusion, depression, and a sense of being absolutely powerless before the onslaught of these symptoms, which went on for months. I was diagnosed and treated by Dr. Lorraine Bonte, who later helped Michael (with his immune deficiency symptoms) to restore his body's defenses after the drugs he had been taking for weeks to destroy the fungal meningitis. This was the "opportunistic infection" that, combined with Kaposi's sarcoma, almost killed him in May of 1985.

I want to emphasize here that I had no known way of "catching" the AIDS virus. I had no contact with Michael until months *after* his hospital stay. I am assuredly heterosexual, and the only contact I had had with Michael in many years was the instance of the funeral of my youngest grandson, Zachary, the previous August, where Michael, on a sweltering day, covered up in a heavy brown suit any evidence of lesions of Kaposi's sarcoma. At that time Michael had been diagnosed with AIDS, but no one knew it, and he was very careful and standoffish with his hugs. He had not yet had the fungal meningitis that led to his first brush with death.

Yet it is both ironic and eerie that at the same time that Michael was going through his life-and-death struggle with AIDS, and all the stresses accompanying that situation, I was going through a devastating divorce; the loss of almost everyone and everything both material and emotional that had been part of my life for eighteen years; the death of my grandson; incredible financial and creative hardships; and finally, the move across country to start over again near three of my four sons and to rebuild and restore my life. I believe that Michael and I, on one level, were going through

the same type of illness at the same time in an eerie symbio-
sis of mother and son *knowing,* at some deep atavastic level,
what was happening with the other, and from *both* our
experiences coming to a much greater love, understanding,
and compassionate regard for one another.

I *did* not and *have* not ever had AIDS (nor do I intend
to), but the powerlessness that accompanies a major life-
debilitating illness *forced* me to affirm and practice my deepest beliefs about God, about healing, about love, about living.
I am well acquainted with the will to live: While Michael
was making his own choice to affirm life, so was I. And
healing our relationship, which had been a source of deep
distress to me, was an affirming process for both of us that
only deepened in love each passing day. At that time I
thought I could not heal the past, wherein Michael *thought*
that I cared more for his stepfather than for him, and which,
in rebellious teenage years, compounded by the rigidity and
indifference of another family member, resulted in his running away from home to live with his father and Nancy.
Scarcely a family in the sixties and seventies did not experience this phenomenon. The tragedy lies in the fact that from
those scars, walls grew up that I was helpless to tear down,
despite all my efforts. Until, that is, both Michael and I
became ill.

Yet Michael and I learned not only to love one another
at a far closer level than we had ever experienced, but from
that joint yet separate excursion into the depths of illness we
were able, each in our own way, to reach out and help
others who were going through the life-and-death issue of
AIDS. AIDS is a family problem. And families can heal.

This may all seem like a curious aside while talking
about the medical aspects of AIDS. But I feel that medical
facts cannot be separated from the whole of the human
being's life; that the shake-up that AIDS generates in the
patient's system brings to the surface all the unresolved

issues that have contributed in some way to the disease. And I also believe that the healing of the AIDS patient, whether he chooses to die quickly, slowly, or not at all at this time, is accomplished within the entire arena of emotions that the AIDS patient is experiencing, *and* that family members are experiencing. There is no longer any doubt in my mind or in the mind of most health professionals that the mind and emotions are a crucial part of healing. Witness the way in which Norman Cousins healed himself in *Anatomy of an Illness* and later, cooperated again with his doctor in recovering completely from a massive heart attack in *The Healing Heart*.

So even as I continue to research and interview those in possession of medical facts, I am reminded again and again of a phrase that my minister, Helen Nairn, used when explaining how healing can work.

"There are the 'facts' about this situation," she would tell me, "and then there is the 'truth' about this situation. If we look only at the exterior evidence, then we cannot change the condition. It is only when we move from the outer 'effect' back to the inward cause that healing can take place."

The "truth" is that you are a magnificent human being, a magnificent expression of God. The "facts" may be that you have chosen this illness to learn something vital. The "truth" is that you are more than a specific collection of symptoms, more than a disease, more than a statistic. To be healed is to learn the lesson and go on. This is not just "pie-in-the-sky" positive thinking. If hope, love, and laughter can heal a prominent man of letters, so the diligent application of the "truth" about you can, at the very least, allow a breathing space wherein each AIDS patient can discover the inner causes that have contributed to the outer disease, change those inner perceptions along with all the medical means at his disposal, and relive his life in a way that honors himself instead of destroying himself.

There are AIDS persons who are living far longer than statistics indicate. Michael and others like him have stories to tell you about just that process in the next chapter. There are also cancer patients who seem free of cancer, as well as heart-attack patients who have strengthened their hearts. There are alternatives to dying, just as there are alternatives to living.

It is worth a serious look at the difference between the "facts" and the "truth," if only because by extending the life span of current AIDS patients, by offering any and all safe adjuncts to current medical treatments (which have not, so far, worked that well), we can then allow time for the AIDS patient to clear up any unfinished business in his life. He can, if he believes entirely and only in the medical prognosis, buy time until a vaccine comes along that will serve as the catalyst (for him) of fighting and curing this dread disease. He can use this time to rethink what his life is all about, and what his death is all about. He can move in some cases from a "victim mentality" to a "victorious" life. And it all has so very little to do with the time span involved, the quantity of years lived, the hours spent and wasted dealing with all the outer "effects" of our culture, instead of and including the quality of time it takes to heal relationships, to clear up the past, to go out of this life in a peaceful way, whenever that may be.

This is not to negate in any way, shape, or form the medical information and medical help available for AIDS patients. We owe it to ourselves to obtain the facts and then make our decisions from the vantage point of the best knowledge and the best help we can find. And so many of the doctors and other health professionals working with AIDS patients give of themselves in selfless, compassionate ways, with a firm understanding of the totality of the person, mind, body, and spirit, and of the ability of the informed AIDS patient to heal himself. This applies to the patient's family and friends as well. Correct information can help one move from the ignorance and fear evidenced by much of the general public's prevailing attitudes to compassion and acceptance. A release of fear invariably leads to a resurgence of love.

Dr. Brooks agrees with this premise. At the time of this writing Dr. Brooks has taken his medical and psychiatric practice to a point where he helps the AIDS patient to deal with considerations of *living*, not *dying*, with AIDS. Dr. Brooks's seminars are entitled, appropriately, "Being Well—Being Gay—AIDS." The following information, written by him, is presented in its entirety with his permission. It is a moving discussion of the factors involved in *living*.

"Being Well—Being Gay—AIDS"

For several years now I have been engaged in the diagnosis and treatment of people with AIDS. Some of the people I am working with are living well beyond the projected expectations made on the basis of current statistics. These people I am referring to have an unusual sense of vitality and robustness way beyond that reported in the medical literature and popular press. When I began to encounter such individuals, I asked myself why some persons with serious illness do so well, while others fare so poorly. My understanding from my training in medicine and biology led me to believe that these kind of differences were the result of genetic and constitutional factors. However, I am no longer convinced this is so. In my opinion, those persons that I see with AIDS who are doing the best are thinking about their situations differently. I want to share with you some of the things I have come to believe about the healing process.

I believe that we live in many different domains simultaneously. Two distinct domains are *physical reality* and our *experience* of our lives. Most people consider their experience of life to be a function of their circumstances. However, this notion is questionable. I believe that our experience of life is more apt to be a function of our interpretation of our circumstances. It is precisely because we live in a sea of language that we fail to notice the power of words. Recently some very sophisticated research involving hypertension has demonstrated that one of the most potent stimulators of elevated blood pressure is human speech, and that one of the best ways to achieve long-term control of pathologically high blood pressure is to modify what has been called the human dialogue. This kind of research expands our concept of the cause of a medical illness to include another dimension of our humanity; in this instance, ourselves as languaging creatures. I have seen a number of people with AIDS create new romantic relationships after their diagnosis, some of them with people who do not have AIDS, by altering the way they were willing to talk about themselves and what was happening to them. I'll have more to say about this in a moment.

I am convinced that well-being resides in our experience of our lives. We can have well-being under any circumstance. Conversely, we can have any circumstance, including wealth and a strong, healthy body, and not experience any sense of well-being. This is a particularly difficult concept for some people to grasp, because, from this point of view, a person with AIDS can have a high level of well-being, as measured by his/her level of active participation in daily living, sense of joy, experience of love, and freedom from negative emotional states and suffering. Many people fall into the trap of thinking that happiness is dependent upon exterior conditions. For them, one must have a particular set of conditions in order to have joy, enthusiasm, or love.

When their conditions are not met, there is no experience of these positive states of mind for them. However, the failure to have these powerful life experiences is not really because of a lack of a particular set of circumstances. It is more truly the result of the way that they have learned to think.

True well-being is an individual choice. It involves a shift of position from considering oneself a victim of circumstances to a creator of experience. This shift takes a tremendous willingness to assume individual responsibility. It literally involves a willingness to experience one's *self* as being powerful enough to be the cause of one's own experience. This kind of talk about responsibility is very difficult, because most people hear blame when the concept of responsibility is used. This is the result of the way we were treated as children. When we were children and did something of which our parents did not approve, their calling us responsible was really a placement of blame. When I see patients who refuse to acknowledge their responsibility, they are really refusing to be blamed. Of course, we can refuse blame, but we cannot abdicate responsibility. We simply are responsible, regardless of whether we are too confused to acknowledge the fact of it or not.

I believe that is why responsible persons with AIDS object so strongly to being referred to as *victims* of AIDS. In their way of thinking, they are *persons* with AIDS, and they are not experiencing their lives as victims of anything. They are creating lives of love, commitment, and with high levels of well-being.

Medicine as a discipline of physical science is powerless to create well-being. The prevention of illness or the eradication of illness is not synonymous with well-being.

In order to include well-being in medical treatment, we have to have an expanded context of medicine. I believe that any intervention which creates a sense of well-being can lend support to healing processes that are going on in the body. The following are components that I believe are necessary to create what I like to call a *healing atmosphere*.

1. Intention. The key to any kind of healing is intention. This has been called the will to live. Without this kind of intention ill persons will not generate the kinds of behaviors that promote survival. I have seen patients who were in the process of dying suddenly create a strong intention to live and, as a result, made miraculous recoveries. I have also seen persons who could have lived a great deal longer, given their current state of health, die prematurely simply because they didn't want to go on any longer.

2. Human Contact and Love. The power of simple human contact and love seem to have been forgotten in this highly technological society of ours. Psychologists have documented the profound effects of lack of touch and love in infants and named this condition the maternal deprivation syndrome. However, to a lesser degree, I think there exists for most persons in the world today an *adult deprivation syndrome*. The results of this are not as obvious, yet I think they are just as serious in terms of health consequences. We all need to be loved and touched. Nowhere is this lack of human contact more apparent than in our modern hospitals, where AIDS patients are more often than not kept in a virtual prison of sensory isolation and needlessly treated as the proverbial lepers of a bygone era. In general, we behave as if these basic requirements for a human existence were somehow dispensable. The truth is that no technological advance will ever replace what is basic to our human nature. I think this is beginning to dawn on most people and underlies many people's anxieties about entering a modern hospital. It's as if our unconscious is creating a warning sign: UNSAFE FOR HUMAN BEINGS.

3. Purpose in Life. The avoidance of death is not a very powerful reason to live, and reasons to live will never be generated by science and technology. A person has the best chance of surviving a serious or catastrophic illness when he/she has *something* he/she considers *worth living for*. Reasons for living come from other domains than science, from those intensely private domains that make us uniquely human. Good physicians know this, although they may not be able to talk about it articulately. All of us in medicine have had the experience of seeing patients who had an overwhelming commitment to something or someone and out of that commitment generated either a cure, or else prolonged periods of improvement beyond what would have ever seemed reasonable under the circumstance. You cannot characterize the kind of experience of being in the presence of an individual so committed.

4. Willingness to Turn Within. The way we view outside authority in the West is truly astonishing. For many of us, if we read it in a book, it's true. If we experience it directly, we doubt it. We have been taught to be profoundly mistrustful of our intuition and basic human experience. Yet the wisdom of the ages has encouraged man to look inward for the answers to life's most difficult questions. I believe that the healing journey begins with a *look inward*, toward ourselves, and a "coming to know" our own truths and healing powers.

I would like to end this short discussion with a brief statement of my position on the matter. I believe that modern medicine has contributed enormous advances to people's well-being. Of this there can be little doubt. However, a large amount of the humanity that is vital to our survival as individuals and as a species has been sadly neglected and ignored by the medical profession. I believe that we are now entering an age of synthesis and cooperation. Just as the superpowers must learn to live together if we are to avoid final extinction in a holocaust, so must medicine learn to live with other disciplines that make a contribution to well-being. Unless physicians humble themselves and learn to respect

other approaches to healing and well-being, they will continue to lose the respect of the very people they are committed to serve. This is a time for a true holism. A time to look
at everything that is of value from any tradition or model.
Science alone no longer makes sense.

Robert N. Brooks, M.D.

I had a unique opportunity to interview Dr. Brooks
about his current practice working almost exclusively with
AIDS patients, the conclusions he has come to regarding
the problem, and the resolution that AIDS brings to a person's life, as well as the part that he, as a medical doctor and
psychiatrist, plays in that AIDS crisis.

For AIDS patients, parents, and friends, his words serve
to put the problem called AIDS into perspective. Indeed,
his insights can help all of us to see more clearly our own
responsibility concerning the life lessons that AIDS brings to
all of us involved with the AIDS phenomenon.

I asked Dr. Brooks five questions. His answers serve to
illuminate the basic issues we are concerned with in this
book; i.e., responsibility, commitment, healing, love. These
basic issues extend far beyond one person's illness, one
family's tragedy. The way we respond to AIDS in our lives,
individually and collectively, reflects our capacity for positive change that can and does extend far beyond us and out
into society as a whole. Here, in Dr. Brooks's own words,
are the healing implications of AIDS.

B.C.M.: What do you think is the major problem AIDS
patients face when healing themselves?

Dr. Brooks: First of all we have to talk about what healing is
and where it takes place. Doctors, patients, modern medicines do not heal. The body heals itself, if it is going to.
There are things that we do to support healing, including

taking advantage of modern medical treatments. In my view there are many nonmedical approaches that can add support to the body's healing processes. I don't think that we need to adopt an either/or model when thinking about what might be of value to a sick person. There are many traditional things that support well-being which are not strictly medical. The problem is that we are usually taught to think in the dialectic or conflict model. This is the model of right/wrong, good/bad, either/or. We have very little experience with cooperation and sharing.

I like to think in terms of creating a healing atmosphere when I think about caring for a sick person. Many disciplines besides standard medicine can contribute to the well-being of an ill person. Patients have been open with me about the things they have done to help themselves, and I have learned a lot by respecting their experience. One of the elements that I think is crucial to creating a healing atmosphere is anything that creates a deep state of relaxation and peace of mind. Meditations and visualizations have the potential to accomplish this. Several of my AIDS patients have told me that they felt their willingness to do this kind of "inner work" was prolonging their lives.

Many of my patients have found that giving up making their lives a survival issue and learning to live moment by moment, finding joy and satisfaction in the *now*, assisted them in finding peace of mind.

B.C.M.: What is the most important contribution you make in your work with AIDS patients?

Dr. Brooks: If I can put a patient in touch with his power to create a sense of well-being in the face of difficult circumstances, then I have contributed a lot. I learned a long time ago that we create the experience of our circumstances. That's a difficult concept to get across most of the time. Many of us have a heavy investment in feeling that we are victims of circumstance, and we all feel justified in our dissatisfaction. However, what I learned is that it's like a game. If our game is to create dissatisfaction, then we will find one thing or another to fret about, worry about, or be upset about. This game costs us. It costs us our peace of mind. This may not seem like much, but it's an enormous price when we are trying to create a mental climate for physical healing to take place. Anger, resentment, guilt, and other negative emotions cost us our peace of mind and our sense of well-being. Ultimately they may cost us our health.

B.C.M.: What would you like to tell AIDS patients and their friends and families?

Dr. Brooks: To love and support each other. That's the most important gift we have to give.

B.C.M.: What are your background credentials, and how did you get into working with gay patients?

Dr. Brooks: I did an undergraduate degree at Stanford University, and medical training at the University of Southern California. Following internship, I practiced general medicine for two years. I completed a residency in psychiatry and practiced psychiatry for five years. I went back to the practice of medicine in a university health service and there began working with gay patients. I discovered that I had a unique combination of skills to deal with the problems of gay men. I opened a private practice devoted to the medical care of gay men. I never expected to be concentrating so much attention on AIDS. My practice opened when AIDS was still a very rare disease. Now most of my work is in some way related to AIDS. I am seeing persons with AIDS or persons concerned about AIDS. Eighteen months ago I started a seminar with a group of other people for the gay community. The seminar is called "Beyond AIDS: Transforming Our

Relationship With Illness." It's quite unusual, something that has never been done before. Many persons with AIDS work with me to create this seminar. We look at many aspects of health care in this program.

B.C.M.: What do you see in the future for AIDS, both positive and negative?

Dr. Brooks: This is the kind of question that I love to answer. As you know, nobody can see the future. However, we can invent possibilities. This is somehow connected with our nature. What I see as possible medically from AIDS is a deep and profound appreciation of the role that our immune system plays in supporting our well-being. I think we will find solutions to many puzzling problems in the area of infections and cancers. A lot of the knowledge that we gain in conquering AIDS will help us treat other diseases more effectively. For AIDS specifically, I think we will find ways to eliminate the virus from the body and develop ways to rehabilitate a damaged immune system. I also think we will produce an effective vaccine that will insure future generations against acquiring the AIDS infection in the first place.

Socially, AIDS will give us the opportunity to clarify our values as human beings. Diseases don't occur in a vacuum; they occur in people who live in social groups. The way we view persons with AIDS presently is colored by many antiquated attitudes and prejudices. We have many outdated notions about gayness and about sexuality in general. We also have profound intolerances to differences. These attitudes and prejudices have the potential to create serious unworkability for the human race. As we approach the twenty-first century AIDS and other major world problems will be resolved within a context which expands our commitments to one another as human beings. There is no space into which to exclude someone who happens to look different or love

differently. We will either be in this together, or else, I
believe, we will all perish. I think God has given us the
choice.

An example might be in the way that insurance companies are behaving. Many of them, not all, have been looking
for ways to identify persons exposed to the AIDS virus for
the purpose of excluding them from the ranks of the insur-
able. This, in my opinion, is a pretty typical and outmoded
way of reacting. I think, as we move closer to a world that
works, we will see approaches that include rather than exclude. In the case of insurance carriers, it would look like
this: Those companies that survived would be the ones that
worked to care for everyone. Somehow economic success
would be tied to service to humanity, not to eliminating
people who need help. I can't describe what those kinds of
institutions would look like, because they don't really exist
yet. However, I think that most biologists agree that a
narrow self-interest is not compatible with long-term survival. For me, the time is at hand for the human race to
examine its commitments to itself. Either we're really committed to taking care of each other, or else forget it.

Psychologically I believe that AIDS will help us to
accept physical illness as a natural phenomenon and not as
an evil thrust upon us. This is a paradox. Just as we work so
hard to treat and cure illness, we must also work hard to
accept the reality of our physicality. I believe that in the
future we will see a dramatic shift of emphasis toward understanding our mental states. In many ways we have been at
war with our biology. Ultimately this does not serve us. I
believe that we will no longer tolerate many of the indigni-
ties that come from trying to prolong physical existence
when it is no longer appropriate. As we deepen our respect
for living, so shall we deepen our respect for dying. We will
stop making a disease out of a natural process. I believe that,
in the future, we will shift the psychological foundation of

our lives from fear and avoidance of so-called negative outcomes to one of self-expression and celebration. We will come to behave more and more in ways that reflect a way of seeing life as a gift.

I also see a deepening appreciation for the spiritual dimensions of our lives. One of the profound things that I have learned from my patients is how important it is that we have a sense of being part of our universe. I call this sense of connectedness *spiritual*, for lack of another term. I know that it is possible to feel like a part of the cosmos, to experience being a part of the whole. This is a deeply healing experience. For me, this experience is very natural and beautiful. Persons who do not allow themselves this experience are usually angry and resentful at not being in control of life's circumstances. For me, it's pretty clear that we each get to create a unique experience of life and to share this with each other. Beyond that, we are mere cogs in the wheel of the machinery of the universe. For me, the universe is perfect. It seems silly to resent being part of perfection. Yet that's the kind of experience we commonly create. However, there are exceptional experiences available to each of us: wonder, joy, celebration, love, to name just a few.

"All your past except its beauty, is gone,
and nothing is left but a blessing."

—A COURSE IN MIRACLES

5

"WHEN I FOUND OUT
I HAD AIDS"

AIDS Patients Tell Their Stories

"AIDS can be a lesson in living, rather than a lesson in dying." That is the startling message in this chapter, which is composed of life histories of AIDS patients (they prefer to be called AIDS *persons*, not AIDS "victims"). The terms *life history* instead of *case history* are used because the people involved, Andrew Hiatt, Louie Nissaney, Susan Roggio, Steve Peters, and all the other AIDS persons I interviewed, are all examples of the principles of love, forgiveness, and responsibility contained in the package called self-healing. At the time I interviewed them, none of these young men (and one woman) knew how long their life span might be.

As one told me jokingly, "I'm healing my life right now in case I step in front of a bus next week."

All of these young people had shifted the focus of their disease into a focus of healing relationships, and from that point of power they were moving on to new challenges that, in many cases, served more than the person involved and indeed reached out into ways to help others, to help the community, even to work on a global level (in commitment, at least) to eradicate the barriers that stand in the way of all healing. As one articulate man said, "Now that I have healed myself, I am ready to work for the healing of the whole planet."

The personal agony these AIDS persons went through, including the grim detailing of the progression of AIDS into a fight between life and death, is chronicled in their own words, through taped and written interviews that capture the roller coaster of emotions that accompany these courageous stories.

At the same time it is important to know that not all of these stories from AIDS patients end in perfect health. Many of these interviews come from a sure place within the individual that states: "My life *is* all about healing. The quality of my life is far more important to me than years measured."

And what of the AIDS patients who cannot tell their stories? What of the thousands who have already died of AIDS and all its attendant complications? What of celebrities like Rock Hudson? What of the young man next to Michael in the AIDS ward when he was treated for fungal meningitis?

Each of these AIDS patients, living or dying, has brought the battle arena of AIDS out of the darkness into the light. Each of these AIDS patients has contributed, in some way, to raising the consciousness of the general public, so that research can be funded to find medical cures. Because of the furor over AIDS as a loathsome plague, discrimination practices against AIDS patients have had to be examined and, in some cases, changed for the better. New legislation, money for research, even the New Morality, in which promiscuity is "out" and "committed relationships" are "in"—all are positive steps that would not and could not be taken if the AIDS problem had not "come out of the closet" to affect not only the immediate family but also, in so very many cases, the general public as well.

I believe that there are no deaths in vain. I believe that

the AIDS patients who have died, and the AIDS patients who have decided to die at this time, those who either do not know or cannot at this time accept such a shift in their belief systems to embrace the possibility of healing, all—*all*! —are valuable to the pieces of the puzzle known as the conundrum of AIDS.

And as a mother, I realize that these words are hollow indeed when it is *your* child who is afflicted, when it is your *loved* one who is dying. My heart goes out to all of you who have witnessed this waste of human potential. I know what loss is all about. But even in those instances in which we lose a loved one, what *can* come out of that "dark night of the soul" is our own healing, our own resurgence, our own regeneration. We must rise from the ashes. To deny our own life because someone we love has gone compounds the loss, multiplies the tragedy. Our own lives are valuable! We have something to share from this tragedy. We have something to give to others. There are no deaths in vain. There are no losses that cannot be overcome. Faith may seem a hollow word at this time, but faith, combined with wisdom and love for the self that is still here on the planet, can move you one tiny step forward each day into your own healing, into your own new beginning, into your own life-affirming, life-caring capacities.

And for those of us who are still living, those with AIDS and those concerned with a loved one's battle with AIDS, here are life-affirming stories that prove that nothing is impossible.

Because Michael has been so dear to me, I am presenting his story first, from a speech he gave at an Intensive Workshop on Healing Support Therapy sponsored by "Expect a Miracle," a San Francisco group based on *A Course in Miracles*. Yet this excerpt is only a small part of Michael's story. As he reached out to help others with AIDS in ever-increasing ways, this speech became his past, while his future became one of ever greater inner healing.

Michael's Story

Hello! My name is Michael Welsch and I am here today to tell you that none of us are *victims*. Yes, that's right. *I am not a victim!* I am still learning, still growing, and still healing my life and all my relationships. That's the way I choose it to be from now on in my life. I hope that by telling the truth about myself and my illness, that this will help you.

I was first diagnosed with AIDS on July 12, 1984. I had just started a job as a concierge at a hotel. I was under lots of pressure, as I had worked sixty hours a week for three years. I always worked and played equally hard. My doctor, Thomas Ainsworth, who had treated me for skin problems, found a purple bruise on my right leg. He referred me to a dermatologist, who did a biopsy. Dr. Ainsworth called me at work the next day and wanted me to come see him.

I said, "You can tell me over the phone. I know what it is."

Dr. Ainsworth said, "No, you don't know what it is. I want you to come see me now."

The doctor told me when I saw him that it was AIDS and that the head doctor at San Francisco General Hospital also concluded it could only be AIDS in the form of Kaposi's sarcoma, a type of skin cancer that appears as a blood tumor. He told me to immediately cut down on my workload and that I had an 80% chance of dying within three years. The percentages went way down after that.

I was devastated. What did I do with this information? Well, the truth was that I didn't tell anybody. In my life I had always been a controller and a martyr and had not allowed people to get close to me. I would always rather be right than happy! I was close to my ex-stepmother Nancy, and I liked the people I worked with, but in all my other family relationships I had played the martyr to the hilt, especially as concerned my father, my mother, and my ex-stepfather. I had been done wrong. I was right, and I was going to handle my life without them. I approached having AIDS with my past patterning—that is, I decided not to share this news or myself with anybody. First, I was totally devastated. Having AIDS frightened me almost to death. I would rather have had any disease rather than AIDS. Not only is AIDS supposedly incurable, but it carries such negative connotations of promiscuity, homosexuality, fear, and confusion. Other people are so afraid of AIDS. So was I. I was so frightened, I carried it around with me for a long time. I even went home to Texas to visit my mother and grandmother and be there for my brother and his wife when their baby Zacky died in August, 1984. Still, I didn't tell anybody.

Finally I couldn't keep it in any longer and decided to tell Nancy (my ex-stepmother), who was really like a mother to me. I went to her house one day and she could tell right away that I was very, very upset. I just started crying, this intense crying, the first time I had allowed myself to cry. I cried forever, it seemed like.

Nancy didn't understand. She thought it was my job or something like that and she kept telling me that "whatever it is, we can get through it."

Then I told her, "It is something so horrible, it is AIDS."

She just couldn't believe it. We both cried and hugged each other and then she told me I could beat it, that I had a choice to live or die.

Well, I dismissed this immediately because I knew she didn't understand what AIDS really was, that this was one disease you can't beat. There is no cure. You get AIDS and then you die. And that's that.

After that Nancy allowed me my space and did her

grieving alone. Later she took me on a trip to Europe (kind of a see-the-world-before-you-die trip). I felt she was doing it because I had AIDS and she wanted to spend more time with me. I was still unaware anything positive could come out of all this. I was very depressed. I fully expected that I was going to die. The trip darkened the sadness in me.

The next thing I did was to insist that Nancy not tell anyone about my disease. I didn't want anybody, not family, not friends, not work, to know. Nancy disagreed but respected my decision.

Why didn't I want anyone to know? I didn't want my family to know because I had so much anger toward some of them and I felt so removed from them. To explain and to clean up and clear out all my feelings from the past was just too devastating. Also, I didn't want people to be sad or to feel sorry for me. I didn't want my workplace to know, because I didn't want them to be afraid or confused. It was such a sensitive issue, and I didn't know how people would react, so I kept all this inside me forever and ever and bottled it all up.

I finally told my friend John, who I had been in a relationship with for three years, but at the time the relationship had become nonsexual. I was very, very frightened to tell him, so I finally took him to a play called the AIDS show, which had little vignettes about different situations AIDS people encounter. Then I finally told him and he was supportive, but what can you say when someone tells you they have AIDS, and *you* have been exposed to it? We didn't communicate very much (I wasn't communicating with anyone then).

So I had a choice of confronting the AIDS issue or not. And I chose not to. Even though lesions were popping up, I felt fine physically, and so I ignored it. I was depressed and into the denial phase of the illness. I didn't reach out to support groups or anyone. I didn't want AIDS to be a reality for me.

Everything seemed okay until May, 1985. I went out with my boss and friends to have a good time. The wine was pouring freely, and as was my habit, I was drinking it freely. The next day I woke up with the worst headache of my life, not a hangover, just unbelievable pain. I had had headaches every single day for two years or so, and I took eight Excedrin a day and sometimes two ten-grain Valiums to get rid of the pain. But nothing helped this, not even a prescription of Demerol my doctor gave me.

So I went to the hospital and they did a brain scan. Negative. Then they did a spinal tap and found I had a fungal meningitis that affects the brain. It was a terrible, terrible disease, and Nancy later told my family that I was out of my head with convulsions, high fever, and incredible pain. At that time I still wouldn't let Nancy tell anyone in my family, and this was very hard on her. She had to sit there and watch me sweat and shake and go out of my head every day. One day she collapsed on the floor outside my room crying and screaming because she couldn't stand to see me in such pain. At one point they started giving me this terrible medicine called Anthoritericine, a poison they use on golf greens to control fungus, putting it in my body through the veins in increased dosages. First, I would have the shakes so bad, the bed would rattle and I would be extremely cold, and then I would become so hot that I would run a 105-degree temperature, and this lasted for six hours every single day for two weeks. Even though I was on morphine and other painkillers, it was horrible (and the only reason I'm even telling you this is because I have come so far, and whatever else I have to tell you about what I went through is just to emphasize how I am now in a better place, a clear, life-affirming place and that the past is over).

Before I checked out of the hospital (I was still going to

be an outpatient for six hours a day every other day for six weeks, with further injections of this poison Anthoritericine), a wonderful, important thing happened to me. I finally allowed Diana, my boss, to visit me in the hospital, not knowing that she had talked to the doctor and knew I had AIDS.

I made myself presentable, and when she walked into my room, she just looked at me and said, "Michael, how *dare* you not allow us in your life to love you?"

And I just surrendered in that moment. I felt a great weight roll off my shoulders, more than I had ever experienced before in my life. I felt I was surrendering to the fact that I had AIDS and that it was all right for people to know that about me and that somehow, some way, everything was going to work out and things were going to be okay. That was the first moment I had any hope whatsoever. As it turns out, I started getting all these little signs from God that I was going to be all right. (And I was not religious or spiritual in any way at that time.)

What I found out was that Diana had been William Calderon's receptionist for five years and practiced self-healing as well. Darcy, my other colleague, had helped her mother heal herself of cancer. So I had a great support system. Diana called William Calderon to find out what I needed to do to beat this. She put affirmations all over my house, and my coworkers took turns taking me to the outpatient AIDS ward for six weeks. So I was getting lots of help.

The AIDS ward was like a horrible negative descent into hell. I would lie there all day with this poison going into my veins. I suffered chills and then sweats. I couldn't eat. I couldn't sleep. Every day I would see all these people come in for shots and they would talk about their terrible AIDS experiences and the next disease they expected to get and about when they were going to die. I hated it!

So Diana gave me a tape to listen to called "Search for

Serenity" from *A Course in Miracles*. It was strange and different, but it really helped me to block everything out. There was a guy in the bed next to me. He was really friendly, but I didn't want to talk to anybody. I didn't want to hear a lot of negativity. But this guy had a tape called "AIDS: A Positive Approach" by Louise Hay, and he wanted to exchange tapes with me. So I did.

When I played that tape, on that day, in that hospital, I felt that the tape was made especially for me at that moment in time. The first time I heard it, I was lying in full view of everyone in the AIDS ward, and I started crying so hard. When it got to the point of picturing the person you resent most in your life, I vomited because it was my father I resented most. Then I realized I had so many ill feelings toward my family for the past and that I had to clear up *all* these ill feelings in order to be at peace.

One of the remarkable signs was that while I was hearing Louise's tape my mother (who, with my younger brother, had recently moved from Texas to Santa Monica), had gone through a similar immune deficiency illness, had healed herself with many alternative methods that would later help me, including a stress therapy training called rebirthing. She was paving the way with methods that would later help me very much. I had really estranged myself from my mother, ever since I left home at fifteen—that was all part of my being a martyr and not being willing to forgive. So here was a person who really loved me and who was going through incredible stresses and changes in her life and who had so much to offer me, had she been aware of my situation.

So I really felt like it was a sign from God that I needed to heal these relationships. What I learned from the tape was that the key to healing is through confrontation and releasing the past. And the only way to do this is to *forgive*! I thought this would be so difficult, forgiving everyone in my family and forgiving the past, but it turned out to be one of the greatest things I have ever done in my life.

After I got out of the hospital I called my family in Santa Monica (my mother, my brother Bob, my brother Bill, and his wife Sharon). Later I called my grandmother and other brother John in Texas. I still denied I had AIDS to them at the time, but I knew I wanted to go to Santa Monica for more healing with Louise Hay's group, because her program was all about nutrition and forgiving, confronting old patterns and releasing the past. I knew I wanted more of that.

One night my brother Bob called me and caught me off-guard. He asked me point-blank if I had AIDS. I allowed myself to cry and I told him the truth. I cried and cried and cried and couldn't even speak. He was so loving and just kept making deep breathing sounds over the phone and helped me to a total release. Right then I decided I was going to have to tell everyone in my family and that I would go to Santa Monica for a month after I finished my outpatient treatment.

Then I told my mother I had AIDS. She was incredibly supportive and loving. It turned out that this experience was about healing our relationship. Everything she was doing in her life had parallels to what was happening in my life. She set up chiropractic and Hellerwork sessions, all kinds of holistic therapy, inner-child-work therapy sessions, and of course, I went to Louise's group. At the same time my grandmother came out from Texas and I had almost a month of daily, intense healing work plus lots of love and support from my family.

When I surrendered to it all and allowed people to love me, I had everything I needed and my life became much easier. And I realized AIDS was a vehicle for me to change my life. Everything was part of this change, from my mother's *A Course in Miracles* group to Louise Hay's Wednesday night group of about one hundred gay men, many with AIDS, who helped and supported one another.

About this inner-child therapy. My mother's friend Steve was in a training program with her (he was one of her teachers), and she brought us together. I was the first person he treated that had AIDS, and now his practice is all about helping AIDS patients to heal themselves. I was really scared about this therapy because I didn't know what was going to happen and so I couldn't control it. But I gave Steve my complete trust and I surrendered and allowed everything that needed to be cleared to come up. It was very intense work. For three hours I allowed all my emotions to come up, great joy as well as tears, anger, and every feeling possible. I got rid of a lot of anger I had toward my mother, and I did a lot of forgiving and releasing and confronted some issues concerning my father, but the real confronting with him came later in a second session. It was as if I cleaned out the past and didn't allow it to direct my life anymore.

At this point the only person in my family (except for my ex-stepfather) who did not know I had AIDS was my father. I had convinced him I didn't have AIDS, and now here was the big confrontation. When I decided to tell him, I was really afraid all day long because I knew the news would be so devastating for him. At the same time I knew I needed to go beyond that point. I needed to say, "Yes, I have AIDS and I'm going to be okay," and convince him of that. I also had to clear up my past relationship with him, my resentment, my hate, my anger at things he had done to me. I didn't know if I could do both at the same time. I didn't know if he could take it, and I knew he needed time to grieve first before all this confrontation, but as I waited for him to come to see me late one night, I got the message that I had to start the healing with him right away, no matter how painful it was for both of us.

So I told my father I had AIDS. He cried. He and I

then proceeded to clear up all the past issues between us, and amazingly he agreed with everything I said.

He kept telling me, "You're right, Michael. I realize that was the wrong thing for me to do, and I'm sorry."

It was cleansing for both of us, and in the end I forgave my father for everything I *thought* he ever did to me, and I forgave myself for holding in that resentment for so long, for allowing it to control me, for allowing it to help manifest this disease called AIDS in me. So I was really trying to love my father for the first time in my life. And it really worked.

You see, that very same day I had a second therapy session with Steve. It was all about my dad, too, but the difference between the sessions was that in this one I was able to turn all the hate and anger I experienced into a wave of love and allow it to go through all my body and really heal me and, from that place inside, allow myself to really love my father.

This was an incredible experience for me, healing that relationship, because in the past my father had always tried to direct and control and manipulate my life, and I rebelled against that. It got to the point where every time he called me, I would think, Oh, God, what do *you* want now? I just never wanted to be around him, because I felt he always wanted something or wanted me to do something for him or told me how to live my life. So now I was able to start coming from love and to realize that it was my choice to be or not be controlled by him. This made me feel so free.

So where am I now? And where is my family now? First, about my family and support system. My mother is writing a counseling book to help parents and loved ones when someone they love has AIDS. My grandmother is writing her thoughts for the manuscript, and the publication of it sounds good. My father is interested in all the research about AIDS, especially the medical discoveries. My brother Bob works full-time for Louise Hay, and Steve (my therapist) is an important part of our lives. My whole family is going to be together at Christmas, and I know even more healing will take place.

I am now facilitating my own Wednesday night group and other groups, using all I have learned about the healing process. What I am learning in those groups about surrendering and letting God take over in the group is also helping me in my life.

I am serving others beautifully and serving myself and really going forward.

What else is true for me? Well, I have changed my nutritional habits. No alcohol, no caffeine, no chocolate, no sugar, no junk foods. And I rarely cheat. I have cleared the junk food out of my system and cleared a lot of junk out of my life. My doctor, my friends, my coworkers, my beautiful ex-stepmother Nancy—are all here for me, as well as my group and all the rest of my family. And I thank God for that.

Sometimes it all gets overwhelming and overpowering for me. Then I think, When is all this going to end? When am I going to be able to stop thinking about AIDS?

There are times when I get scared and despairing. Then I realize that I am still in the midst of my healing, that I am in the perfect place for me, working with people I love. That's when I realize that control is not what it's all about. Healing and love and surrendering to God is what it's all about. I needed to wake up, I needed to understand that the patterns that I had created in my life were not serving me. I needed to wake up spiritually and emotionally and mentally and physically, and I have done that and am still doing that. I've been able to share myself. I've been able to heal old relationships that were bringing me down and keeping me apart from people I love and who love me. I've been able to release patterns that just didn't serve me or anyone else.

My life is not over yet. I have a lot of things I'm going to learn in this lifetime. I'm excited about this opportunity to learn to love myself and others more deeply and fully than I ever have.

I really thank God that I've had this chance to wake up to my own life.

—Michael Welsch
November, 1985

After Michael first spoke out about his experience, he was able to reach out to many other AIDS patients. He had support groups in his home, a telephone counseling support network, and worked as a facilitator with "Expect a Miracle" (whose techniques, based on *A Course in Miracles*, along with Steve Parrish's inner-child therapy work and Louise Hay's support groups, will be profiled in later chapters). All this was in addition to his regular job at a hotel.

Michael had several setbacks during that time. But each time he confounded medical opinion either by recovering quickly or, in one case, detailed in a later chapter, proving X rays and a diagnosis of pneumocystis carnii to be incorrect and walking out of the hospital instead of into it. He continued to rebuild his relationships and to work with transforming processes. He was careful to eat correctly, get plenty of rest, and to follow the guidance of the health professionals in his life.

And what did Michael want to do for the rest of his life? "Help other people," Michael said without hesitation. "And be happy. I want to reach out to others like they reached out to me. I feel that I was given a second chance at life, and I want my life to be one that has meaning. I want to be of service by changing my life and communicating that change to others.

"I have learned to celebrate life, instead of living in death."

"The most important thing I have learned is that one of the prime elements of human uniqueness is the ability to

create and exercise new options." So says Norman Cousins
in "Survival as an Option," *New Realities* magazine, January/
February 1985.

I heard those same words echoed and paraphrased time
and time again as I interviewed AIDS patients who had
seized new options for their lives, using AIDS as a catalyst.

Michael is not the only person who chose a life sentence
instead of a death sentence. I sent out a questionnaire to
almost a hundred people with AIDS who were involved in
healing themselves in some form or another through support-
group work, intensive retraining through psychological and
spiritual holistic healing methods of all kinds. All of these
people had contracted some form of AIDS, whether pneumocystis carnii, Kaposi's sarcoma, fungal meningitis, lymphoma, or a combination of symptoms. In each case some
type of opportunistic infection had appeared. They were
then diagnosed by medical doctors as having AIDS; went to
the hospital; usually went through a death-encountering experience; made the decision at some level of their being to
live; searched for ways to implement that decision in all
areas of their lives; found the help they needed; turned their
lives around in some way, shape, or form; began clearing up
the past; and then, in some fashion, reached out to help
others for whatever length of time they felt they had remaining, from sixty days to sixty years.

Many of these AIDS persons had friends who had died
of AIDS. They had, in some cases, watched these friends
die. Yet each of these living AIDS persons were living
joyfully and intensely. I wanted to know why. What were
the factors involved in wellness instead of illness?

I set up interviews in person and on the phone, with
another ten or so AIDS patients who were in remission (or
so they were told by their doctors). None of them knew how
long they would live. All of them, however, were determined to use their time to extend themselves outward in

some meaningful way. They wanted their lives to count for something.

I chose two additional stories from the many they told me. May these intimate glimpses into others' lives help all who read of their lives—lives, not deaths!

This is not a scientific sample. Obviously I could reach only a fraction of AIDS patients, and of those, only those still living and still immersed in the healing process. And so they are—immersed in life as they never were before. The stories are radically different. The insights, the experiences, are individual. Yet everyone I heard from had common denominators—that is, they had chosen to live by choosing to change their lives in dramatic, inspiring ways. They had chosen to use the remainder of their lives in healing, loving ways. They had chosen to go beyond what they thought they were previously to what they now knew they could be. Without limitation, without equivocation, they had all chosen to heal their relationships.

Susan's Story

Women do get AIDS. Susan did, and she began a path of intense self-questioning into "the dark side of me," to find out how to heal herself and how to be happier.

"I've always been self-destructive," she admitted with the characteristic honesty of the AIDS survivor. "The difference now is that I'm not blaming others. I've always," she went on, "played devil's advocate when it came to myself. Now I'm 'playing' at a whole new level."

For Susan the path of healing has been one of intense self-questioning for many years. An attractive, slender woman in her thirties from a prominent family in the Southeast, Susan and her doctors are baffled as to the manner in which she contracted AIDS. While she had been an intravenous drug user at one time, she had also been in a variety of drug rehabilitation and support-group programs for fifteen years. In fact, she stopped all drug use in 1977. Her doctor insists she must have been in an incubation period all those years, an incredible statement that gives the lie to the often repeated words, "Just stop what you're doing and you won't get AIDS or pass AIDS along."

Since many doctors are still at a loss to explain exactly how the AIDS virus incubates and for how long (at least at the time of this book's publication), I will leave it to Susan to tell her own story, in her own words, of her battle with AIDS, the healing crisis she went through, and her continuing search for healing by alternative methods.

According to Susan, there was no other opportunity, except for her drug use in the 1970s, for her to "catch" AIDS. She is happily married, and her husband has been tested for the HTLV-III virus. He does not have AIDS. They have always had a normal, healthy sex life. In fact, Susan told me that even after the AIDS diagnosis they continue with their sexual activities together, now following the AIDS Project, Los Angeles's guidelines for "safe sex." Susan and her husband have no children of their own, although there are grown stepchildren from his previous marriage. Naturally her husband is having a difficult time adjusting to Susan's illness. Yet he is faithful and committed to their relationship. They are both receiving a lot of therapeutic support and will continue to do so.

Susan is less optimistic about her mother's continuing grief over Susan's illness. While her mother is understanding and supportive, she is going through intense pain and difficulty adjusting to Susan's AIDS diagnosis. (At least, according to Susan's perception of her mother.) Susan feels that her mother is in the denial phase of the illness—that is, she can't really believe Susan does, in fact, have AIDS. Susan feels that her mother doesn't believe that Susan will get well, even though she told Susan's doctor at one point, "You're wrong when you say my little girl is going to die." For Susan's mother the road is triply hard. She has already lost one child and her husband to cancer during the last few years. She has dealt with death again and again. It is understandable that she often asks herself the question, "Why me?" There are no answers to this question for her. Yet it is important to note that as Susan continues to go through therapeutic sessions such as rebirthing (inner-child therapy), she is becoming more aware of her mother's feelings and more compassionate concerning her mother's emotions. As Susan's perceptions change, so are her relationships changing, a phenomenon noted often within the families of AIDS persons.

Susan shared with me the details of her illness:

"I was diagnosed with pneumocystis carnii in May 1985. What happened was this: Six months before the diagnosis, I contracted severe bronchitis and was in bed for a month. Even though I had worked diligently for years to clear up my allergies and my bronchitis, the lung problems just seemed to keep coming back. I was weak and sick for months, lethargic, no energy, scared and depressed. Then I got pneumonia. I was taken to the hospital where I was given strong antibiotics for twenty-four hours, but I just got worse and worse in the hospital and finally had to be moved into intensive care. I was there in intensive care for three days and in the hospital for two weeks. The doctor did a biopsy and found out that I had AIDS. The pneumocystis was so severe that the doctor told my husband and my mother that I would die within a few days, right there in the hospital. He told them that there was no hope at all and that they needed to prepare themselves for my death.

"My mother told the doctor, 'Don't you dare tell Susan

that she has AIDS!' She didn't want me to be scared. She didn't want me to give up. But I was already scared and fighting for each breath. I couldn't talk at all. I had to write notes to communicate with the doctor, even though I could hardly hold a pen to write. But I was stubborn. When the doctor wanted to put a tube in my throat and put me on a respirator, I wrote a note to him that said, 'Let me fight this without the respirator. No tubes, please! If I can't fight it, then put me under.' The pain of gasping continually for each breath was intense. So the hospital used a heavy oxygen mask instead. The oxygen level in my blood was extremely low. I remember that there were lots of intravenous hookups, too, hookups everywhere in me. I also had a lot of rashes, like fungal rashes. And all the medicines made me sicker and sicker. I had such high fevers that the nurses covered me with ice packs. I remember a huge refrigerator at the end of my bed and the ice packs they would take out of it and put all around me. But nothing seemed to bring my fever down. Yet I remember feeling unbelievably cold. Even my bones were cold. Every fifteen minutes they would come in and test me to see if I could still breathe. I was at the very edge of death. I knew it. They knew it. I remember at one point fighting with a dark, cold presence that wanted to take me away. This presence was real to me. It was an energy presence, cold, evil, malicious. I remember fighting with this presence, determined to live, determined not to give in, determined to win in this battle with this cold heaviness that seemed to be all around me. Finally I seemed to feel a tube of light all around my body, and I relaxed into that light, and the cold "thing," it was *death*,—I knew it!—went away. Then I finally slept and was warm. I turned it all around and came out of it, this battle with death. *I refused to die*.

    "After it was all over the doctor told me, 'I don't believe it. You're not supposed to be here.' And I told him, 'Well, I am here. And I intend to stay here.' I really think that I lived because I just love spiting people and getting the best of people." Susan laughed. "I guess you could say that I was always a rebel."

I asked Susan why she thought she got the disease, beyond the obvious medical facts.

She answered: "I had to learn to look at my past patterns of living and behaving. That's the crux of the matter. You see, I always had lung problems. According to this intensive workshop I am in now (while I was interviewing her), lung problems represent an inability to take in life. I have had asthma and bronchitis since I was very young. In fact, I almost died several times as a child. There was an enormous amount of stress within my home when I was born. Although I was a wanted child, the last of six children, and often told that I was a special blessing for my parents, I was conscious of that stress within the home. My father was going through a rough time when I was born. I don't know all the specifics, just that he was a well-to-do contractor involved in lengthy legal trials of a political nature. It was kind of like Watergate. All I know is that I have always been a fighter. Just like my dad. I remember, when I was in the hospital, I made the decision to fight back with everything I had. I didn't know I had AIDS at the time. I'm glad I didn't know. Because the truth is, there was no instant in which I ever decided to die. I chose to fight back against all odds. In this way I am very much like my father. Yet at the same time I realize that I have always had a self-destructive side. I have been told, 'You have courted death all your life.' And so, when I came to this intensive seminar, I had to face that question again and again, and I was asked it over and over. 'Why do you think you got AIDS?' And I had to look deeply within myself, into my character and personality and background, and then take total responsibility for my life, and almost death. I had to ask myself: 'Who are you, Susan? What are you learning from all this? How is the future going to be different from the past?' So I looked within myself and I didn't like what I saw. I realized that I didn't feel good about myself. Or at least I didn't until AIDS came along to wake me up to myself. And I realized that not feeling good about myself is the connection between myself and the gay men who have AIDS. Some of them, though not all, are also heavy drug users and alcoholics. We're often compulsive, excessive people. It's the addict personality. I found out in this seminar that none of us like ourselves. None! We all hated looking at ourselves.

"Specifically I felt like I had screwed up my life long before I got AIDS. I had a nice life-style and a good husband and no apparent problems. Yet the core thought I held was this: 'Everything I turn to in life doesn't work out.' I was full of resentment and bitterness because of a business situation I had been in for over a year. I had invested my husband's money with a friend (or so I thought). This person was an alcoholic and a drug user. The business situation got worse and worse, and the money just dwindled away. I held all this information within me, hysteria mounting within me for over a year. I couldn't tell my husband of my bad judgment. I couldn't handle the pressure of the failing business. I was having tremendous fears and lots of nightmares. I couldn't see my way out of the whole mess. I didn't see how I could tell the truth about the whole business situation. Then I got sick. The whole situation was a trigger point for my illness.

"Now I am finally telling the truth. I told my husband about this failure of mine (the business deal) on my birthday. That was a turning point for me. Now there are lots of turning points for me. I am finally learning to face my fears. I am learning to face myself. In this seminar I learned that when the fear and negativity get to be too much for me, I can just tell my fear to go outside and wait for me. Meanwhile I meditate. And then I take constructive action. What eliminates fear is doing. And what I am doing is learning to love myself. I am opening that door more and more. And when I really believe that I love myself, then I can help others."

Susan paused for breath, then went on earnestly. "I really believe that God has given me AIDS for a reason. There's a lesson behind all of this. My meditations tell me that AIDS is a long-term teacher for me. I can teach by doing. I can teach by example. This all makes me stronger so I can help others. Yet the truth is, I have this fear of going public, because of my family. I am confronting this fear in two ways. I am coming out in the AIDS videotape documentary (*Doors Opening: A Positive Approach to AIDS*), and I am telling my story to you. I realize that I've only just begun to heal myself and to be true to myself, even after fifteen years of therapy. I had to get AIDS to really learn to face myself. I had to go to death's door in order to find out how much I want to live. I had to almost die before I could learn to love myself. And I've only just begun!"

I asked Susan about any differences she may have felt being the only woman with AIDS in an intensive workshop with gay men who have AIDS.

Susan told me: "I am different from the gay men who have AIDS. Obviously, just by being a woman and heterosexual. Some of my concerns are different. My orientation toward life is different. Yet my gay friends have touched my life in moving ways. I am not uncomfortable with them or with the gay life-style. It is easy for me to care for my gay friends without fear. They, in turn, seem to accept me. I guess that's really the whole key. As I grow more accepting of others, others grow more accepting of me. Acceptance is just another word for love."

Steve Peters's Story

For Steve Peters, a gay minister with AIDS who works in a traditional church with a traditional view of Christianity, acceptance takes on ramifications that few of us will ever have to deal with.

Here is Steve Peters's story in his own words.

"I had been sick from June of 1982 with symptoms of AIDS. Looking back, I believe I caught AIDS in the spring of 1981. I had Kaposi's sarcoma and lymphoma (my lymph system wouldn't work). In May 1984, my doctor told me that I was a walking time bomb. In October 1985, my adrenal glands failed. Even as I talk to you, I have just gone through a severe infection and am now on an experimental drug called Seramin. I feel that I am now creating more favorable conditions for the drug to work. There are very few side effects for me, and this is unusual. I now feel that I am in remission. Only time will tell. The doctor told me at one point that he was amazed at my recuperative powers. He told me: 'You and your condition are a deep mystery to me. Scientific testing now shows no evidence of AIDS at this time.'

"What does this tell me? It is my personal belief that God is giving me enough time to do what needs to be done in my life. I have a strong faith in God and His plan for my life.

"My background, which includes many years of spiritual studies and a master's degree in theology, and my ministerial post (I am a minister at the Metropolitan Community Church in the San Fernando Valley), gives me a perfect opportunity to continue my spiritual work within the context of AIDS because my primary outreach is to the gay community. I use traditional Christianity as the base of my ministry, but I feel I have taken my work beyond that. I have studied the works of Steven Levine, Ram Dass, and others who work in a spiritual way with the dying. I continue to study spiritual disciplines. At the same time I have preached again and again about being a Christian with AIDS. I recently spoke on the PTL Club (a cable Christian television show) and I was able to reach 10 million homes to tell everyone that yes, I am a Christian with AIDS and a minister with AIDS, and that my deepest beliefs about Christianity have helped me to survive, have helped me to believe in healing for myself and others. I tell people everywhere that AIDS is not a punishment, not God's wrath. It's just a disease. Since I feel that what I have learned I can't keep to myself, that I can't keep healing unless I give it away, I continue to speak out."

I asked Steve to tell me exactly what he shares with other Christians who may hold different beliefs about homosexuality, Christianity, and AIDS. What happens, for example, when deep-seated fundamentalists hear Steve's story?

"Strangely enough, they do listen. Some even seem impressed by my truth and love. I use Biblical passages that deal with this specific issue—homosexuality—Leviticus and Romans. If they, in turn, try to quote scripture to me, I can quote the Bible back to them. Of course, there are times when I do run across people who won't listen, who won't hear me, whose minds are closed to anyone whose beliefs are different from theirs. I know then that I can't change anyone. I can't change their feelings or their entrenched belief systems. I don't even try. I leave them in their space and bless them on their way. I feel at peace about where I am now and where I am going and what I have to say. You see, before I got AIDS, I was trying to minister, trying to help others, but I really couldn't. I started waking up when AIDS hit. To me AIDS is an incredible gift of awakening. It has helped me to realize my own sense of self and what I have to give. So now I tell others, like I did on the TV, the truth of my experience of awakening. Through sharing my story I am able to communicate effectively. People I share with have to stop and think about AIDS. Sometimes I awaken others through confrontation. I believe that I force others to think, to really think, to examine their own prejudices and to examine their own relationships to God and being a Christian. I am still a Christian; I am a man, a minister, who has AIDS, that's all. I do a lot of sermons on all the implications of being a Christian with AIDS. I believe that this has helped many people to reexamine their beliefs. One of my sermons deals specifically with the issue of fear. This is a big one for anyone who has AIDS.

"Another wonderful thing that has happened, as I learn each day of the gift that AIDS has brought into my life, is that my relationships have changed. My love has changed and become an impersonal love. I have all kinds of loving friends around me now, and I am able to reach out to others, many others, not as partners in a sexual relationship but as friends. Before I got AIDS, I often felt that nobody loved me. Now there's not as much need for one person; I can reach out to so many friends. I feel that I am now in a singular position. Instead of walking two by two like Noah's Ark, my love is there for the whole world. I am, in essence, loving out into the world, helping people I may never meet in person. I feel that God has told me that I can't keep love until I give it away. In fact, what I feel is that I, Steve Peters, am now scared into *life* instead of being scared to death. And I thank God for this every day."

While each of these AIDS persons are unique in that they have all truly used AIDS to reach new levels of understanding, acceptance, and love, there are many other AIDS people out there who are going through their own Gethsemanes. None of these people know how long they will live.

Do any of us? But they are all survivors in the truest sense of the word, using their time to live in the best way they know how, and with a level of trust that is remarkable.

How many more persons like these are out there? It's anybody's guess at this point. The numbers change daily on those who choose to come out and tell their stories, who choose to go to any and all lengths to heal themselves, who choose to use AIDS as a vehicle for psychological and spiritual growth.

Their numbers are growing. While these three AIDS persons, and the others I interviewed, are still in the minority, their message is clear. "AIDS can be a gift that awakens you to life, instead of a death sentence."

> "When I am healed, I am not healed alone."
> —A COURSE IN MIRACLES

═6═ "WHEN I FOUND OUT MY LOVED ONE HAD AIDS"

Parents and Others Tell Their Stories

A Grandmother's Thoughts On AIDS

I am Michael's grandmother, and in 1985 I learned that Michael had AIDS.

The knowledge hits you like a jab in the stomach. You feel with your heart, while your mind rejects the news. It can't be! It can't happen to us! Michael is not! No—could not—would not—join that category of people most susceptible to AIDS! Thus I told myself, rejecting fiercely the possibility, and yes, the probability, that Michael would, of course, get AIDS.

Every thought of Michael, for the past ten or twelve years, has been love wrapped in regret. Family troubles had put him in another sphere of living, away from the family hearth but not outside our love. I felt sometimes that no matter how much I called him, no matter how many times I told him I loved him, that it would roll off his shoulders like dandruff, brushed away by those barriers we, as a family, had built up during the years. Those years were his most important ones, perhaps, his years from fifteen to twenty-five. A barrier as wide as a mountain reared between us. We tried to climb over it, but it seemed impossible to feel really close to Michael, as if anything we said would be accepted but not really warmly received. It is a heartbreaking feeling when you have an idea that nothing will ever reach his heart again.

Then a miraculous few days came along when we made possible a trip to see him. We were suddenly and beautifully together, as if the long years had never been. We laughed over incidents in his childhood. I think he was surprised, and pleased, to find I had held him in memory for so long, steadfast in my love, if not my understanding. We played in the city of San Francisco. We shared food and sights, memories and joy. We told each other things we hadn't dared to say before that time. It was a comfortable time together, a happy time, that helped to heal the barren years preceding that week.

I even met his stepmother for lunch, shared laughter and good talk, neither of us rehashing some bitter words of the past. I was even able to tell her, from my heart, how much I appreciated her loving mothering of Michael in the years apart from our family. It was not hard to do. The closeness Michael and I had suddenly gained made it just the most natural thing to hug Nancy and tell her how much her love had meant to Michael, and still did.

Maybe I knew, in my deepest heart and mind, that Michael was a homosexual, and that Michael might have contracted AIDS. His face was not smooth as it used to be; a spreading myriad of bumps was there on the surface. But he seemed well and healthy, and I put the thoughts aside, although at one point, when he had to slow down, while I, at almost seventy, could still keep going, gave me an anxious moment.

So, it was only a month later that he called me from San

Francisco and told me, in a calm manner, that he had AIDS and had just recovered from a deadly three weeks in the hospital, while I thought he was on a planned visit to New York.

What do you say at a traumatic time like that? I think I was quiet for a moment while I tried to collect my thoughts, tried to answer calmly, to make him know that I loved him. Then, afterward, the tears came. My grandson had just told me he had a death threat hanging over him, a dread disease that not only killed without mercy, like cancer, and without even that hope, but also a disease fraught with social stigma. Some griefs you can share with other members of the family, with friends. That makes it possible to pray together, to share the fear and the coming of death into your midst. This news I could not share with anyone, except the few in the family who had been told of it. How could I face friends and say, "My grandson has AIDS," when I knew they would come back with either the words or the unspoken thought, "Is he a homosexual?"

I had a nephew who died last winter of a pulmonary infection that the doctors said was incurable. He, too, was a homosexual, although neither my sister (his mother) nor his brother told me. I am positive it was AIDS he had. He was not my favorite nephew. We didn't see eye to eye on many things. But I was impressed by the calmness of his arrangements for his own death, not denying it, and his well-thought-out plans for his own cremation and the disposition of those ashes. When I spoke with him the day before he died, I think I liked him better than I ever did. There was a spark of courage in his eyes that made platitudes and sympathy out of place.

And so it was with Michael. He was filled with hope, so strong that you could feel it in his presence. A group of family members was together for a week in the summer of 1985, and Michael's smile and his attitude of hope and certainty of beating this disease set the tone for the whole week. I could cry into my pillow at night. I could pace a track on the rug when I couldn't sleep. I could pray for recovery, for strength, for comfort, for understanding. But I could not, when I looked at Michael, give in to the thought of sure death for him, because of his positive attitude. It was an aura that surrounded him. Most of all, his joy at being close and in mutual understanding, at last, with members of the family, mainly his mother and me, permeated all the times we had together.

It is a paradox that when something tragic, or even shameful in the eyes of the world, attacks your own loved ones, it turns the tables on your thinking and your understanding. You have to open up a little; you have to really look at the issues at hand, not just with your heart but with every atom of wisdom you hope you have. My whole being recoils from the idea of homosexuality. I do not consider myself a sanctimonious, Bible-toting person. I am a Christian, which means I try to follow Christ's ways. I *know* he walked with lepers and had compassion on all afflictions and the people who bore them. For Christ epitomized the love of God, which is ever-reaching, never-failing. But God set up principles of behavior among men, which makes homosexuality beyond the pale of moral law. No matter how the *times* have changed, no matter how loosely a lot of people consider adultery these days, the mere acceptance of it doesn't change God's laws. No matter how much I have loved Michael, no matter how close we may have been in love and understanding, I can never accept the fact that he or any other of my grandsons have chosen this kind of life. And now that AIDS is taking its greatest proportions of lives from among the homosexuals, I cannot see how anyone could choose, with open eyes, this pathway to destruction.

In my view, the *only* way at this time to conquer the growing epidemic of AIDS is to *quit passing it along*!

Michael became very active in working with others who had AIDS, giving hope and a helping hand in the upward climb to understanding this disease that frightens us so much. My daughter also is giving so much of herself to the support groups and the education of people who have AIDS persons in their families. I am so proud of them. I want to be a part of this movement too. I want to help. I want other grandparents out there to know there are millions who are facing the news and don't know where to turn. And I say to them: Turn first to God in prayer. It is the strongest weapon we have, and we do not ever know of all the miracles prayer has wrought. But do not give in to grief, because there *is* hope. Don't recoil from that grandchild who has contracted AIDS. He is still the same little boy (just grown-up now) who came running joyfully into your arms to show off his Superman suit, the same little boy who used to play games with you, whose dimples and shining dark eyes made any day brighter and more blessed.

Be glad that you have a little time to understand and give a greater measure of yourself to your loved one with AIDS. I find I have gained a greater capacity for love and understanding through Michael; and I am proud to be Michael's grandmother.

Michael's grandmother has had the courage to express her feelings about Michael's illness. Your own feelings, your own background, may be different. You may feel as strongly as Michael's grandmother about the moral and religious issues concerning AIDS, or you may disagree violently. One thing is clear, though. You must go through your feelings about AIDS no matter how painful the process, no matter how long it takes. For when someone you love has AIDS, there is no place to run, no place to hide. We survive and help our loved ones. Or we go under.

Norman Cousins, in the same *New Realities* article quoted

earlier, tells us that the single most important lesson he has learned is that "human capacity is what it has to be."

I am reminded daily that all of us who surround the AIDS survivors have to go through an individual, intense confrontation with life and death. Go through it we must. Go through it we do. Then and only then can we come to terms (sometimes kicking, fighting, and screaming all the way) with our own capacity for survival, our own ability to change, to grow, to heal, to accept, to love. We become aware of our own capacities for caring and our own strengths in a crisis situation.

When someone you love has AIDS, there is always fear, always! There are also anger, guilt, grief, all the so-called "negative" emotions of being a human being in a shocking situation. This is normal and natural. It is only when we refuse to move past the initial shock that we stay stuck. No one can rescue you from this place. No one can move you past the fear into the clearing. No one, that is, but you. Again and again I have had to tell myself, "You get through by going through. Your faith may lead the way, but you must take the steps."

As I wrote these words an amazing example of synchronicity came into play.

The phone rang. The person on the other end of the phone was unknown to me. The scared, tension-filled, close-to-tears voice was not.

"I am a mother whose son has AIDS, and I was told to call you. I don't want anyone to know that I'm calling. So please don't call me. My husband and I have a business in our home and we can't let his secretary know. Good help is so hard to find. We can't let anyone know. It would wreck everything." She paused to take a breath. "Why I called you I don't know. I was given your name and phone number. I know you can't help me. I know you can't. No one can help me. It's just impossible. My life is over. My son's life is over. It's just impossible."

She started to hang up even as I began gently explaining that I wanted to talk with her, get to know her, share with her the experiences she was going through.

I reached out across the line to try to break through the barrier in some way. "I know what you're going through. And it doesn't have to be that way. Please, let's talk. Anything you say will be held in confidence. I'm here to help, and if you want to share your experiences of your son's illness with me, and with other mothers, you will be protected, anonymous."

"No! I can't! Don't call me. I don't want to talk. I don't want anyone to know." She hung up before I could reassure her further.

Fear is a powerful deterrent to healing. For many of us the initial shock of learning that someone we love has AIDS sends us into a panic state. The connotations of it all! The social stigma, the unpalatable sexual overtones, the anxiety and helplessness over a seemingly irrevocable diagnosis; all these factors, combined with fierce, underlying anger (I know that one well!) can render us impotent, helpless. "I don't want to know. I don't want anyone else to know." Living in fear and anger, we slam shut the door to other possibilities. For some parents the AIDS diagnosis closes this door completely on any further communication between parent and child. But for most the love that exists underneath the shock and the anger explodes the family into an emotional whirlpool of feelings that cannot be contained. As one AIDS parent told me wryly, "There's nothing like a death sentence to clear up your life."

Fear is not limited to parents. Friends fall away, lovers run, bosses and coworkers sometimes disappear, insurance companies cut you off, ambulances refuse to pick you up and take you to the hospital, dentists refuse to work on you, sometimes even funeral homes refuse to handle the body of an AIDS patient—the list goes on and on. It is no wonder that the anxious mother on the phone screamed at me, "It's just impossible."

And it doesn't have to be that way! For every anguished closing of a door there are new doors that open to healing for everyone who associates with the AIDS person who has decided to live. Even for those AIDS patients that die, many choose to "clean up their act" with their family and friends before they go on into another dimension. And you, as a parent, as a friend, as a coworker or health professional, are as involved in that "clearing up and clearing out" as the AIDS patient is.

A Course in Miracles states: "When I am healed, I am not healed alone." I have found this to be true for me in my life. However long the length of life, the AIDS person and all those around him have a magnificent opportunity to live more fully, more lovingly, more honestly, more in the present moment, than ever before. AIDS won't go away because we refuse to talk about it. AIDS won't go away as we ignore our feelings. That's denial. But by using the fact or condition of AIDS happening within the family structure as an opportunity for healing and closeness, even the death of someone we love can have meaning.

This is the message I received in various forms when I sent out a questionnaire, supplemented by personal interviews with those family members, friends, lovers, coworkers, and healing helpers who were connected with someone who had AIDS. What I found was an outpouring of emotions and some unique insights.

Here is the questionnaire and a sampling of the answers.

1. What were your initial reactions upon learning that _____ had AIDS?

"I was in shock. I walked around for days, angry, angry, angry."

"I took him in my arms and we both cried, the first time we had held each other and the first time we had cried together since he was a little boy."

"I hate the illness, but I love my son. That's all I can say."

"I told him that I loved him and that we could beat it together."

"I decided that I was going to be with my friend all the way, no matter what it took."

"I didn't want anyone to know. I carried it (the AIDS death sentence) around with me for ages before I broke down and told the rest of the family."

"I didn't buy it. I told my friend that he could turn his disease around; really, that he could turn his life around by owning the responsibility that he created the disease, thus he could create health. This is hard love, but it works."

2. How did the AIDS person react to you and to others? Describe reactions of family members, friends, doctors, etc. Describe your reactions to their reactions.

"I was having lunch with Jeffrey and three other men who had AIDS. When I relayed the message that he could heal himself, the other three men were extremely resistant. Jeffrey alone was willing to consider the possibility of getting well. He went through the usual anger, confusion, fear, but within a few weeks of working together on attitude change, he turned his health around and has no sign of ARC."

"I told Michael how angry I was at him for keeping the diagnosis to himself. I told him, 'How dare you not let me into your life to love you!' I knew he could be healed and I communicated that information to him in every way I knew how. I put action behind my beliefs."

"I told him that I was there for him and that he still had a job, so that he had better get well and get back to work where he was needed."

"My mother was really fearful about letting anyone else in the family know. She had to work through her own anger and grief before she told anyone. When she told some, but not all of the people in the family, they, too, had to decide whether or not to tell others. One family member didn't want to tell her kids because it might traumatize them to know that their cousin had AIDS. I didn't agree with that decision, but it wasn't my decision to make."

"Everyone in this one family knew except for the mother of the AIDS person. She was told he was dying of leukemia. Even when she came out from the East to visit with him, no one told her the truth. It was as if it was all right for him to die but not all right for him to have AIDS. I thought this was criminal."

"It really hurt my son when a family friend was fearful about having him stay in her apartment while she was gone. She was afraid she might get AIDS from touching the surfaces he had touched. But she went ahead, anyway, and shared her apartment, which, considering her fear, was an act of love."

"All I could think of was that I had to get all the facts, all the research, talk to everyone I knew, every expert I could find, anywhere, and really find out what was going to happen to my son. But all I found out was so negative. I'm still in a depression, a severe depression, trying to sort it all out."

"I want to believe that my son will live, but I don't really believe it. I'm bracing myself, just waiting for him to die."

"I want to help in any way I can, but I feel helpless. Everyone I talk to just looks at me as if I were a leper. They're sorry for me, but I know they're thinking 'How could you have a son who would do this to you, get this terrible, loathsome disease.' It's as if I'm the carrier, not him."

"My boss came into my work area and told me he had heard that I volunteered at a center that helped AIDS persons. He asked me if I touched any of them. I told him yes, and that I hugged them too. I tried to explain what it was all about. He fired me. He told me he couldn't have anyone around the beauty shop who had been exposed to AIDS patients. It was the best thing he could have done for me, because now I'm really doing what I want to do, helping AIDS patients through my new job."

None of these reactions are good or bad. They are just normal, human reactions to a crisis of this magnitude. It is natural for people to be afraid or angry or guilty or sad or numb or to experience any other emotion, including the emotions of courage, love, and acceptance. There is also, quite often, a fierce determination to change what is happening. In some instances people have chosen to be a part of the process the AIDS person is going through.

What I got out of the answers to my questionnaire, unscientific as it was, was that people are resilient, far more than I had ever imagined. I understood that people are entitled to their feelings, whatever form these feelings take, and that those same feelings will change as time goes on and the person involved learns more about AIDS and what can and cannot be done about it.

To that end, support groups can be very helpful for the AIDS person and his family. In some support groups all is sweetness and light (a welcome change from the death prophecies the AIDS family has previously encountered). In others it's confrontation: "Clear up the mess in your life and you won't die, and/or clear up the mess in your life before you die." Some support groups exist by playing "ain't it awful."

Others are there to ease the dying process. Some are political, dealing with legislation, ending discrimination against AIDS patients. The family of the AIDS person may have to explore several different modes of dealing with the AIDS crisis in order to find out what works for them at various stages of their involvement with AIDS.

I have been involved with several dedicated groups who are mentioned in succeeding chapters. What I found out as I visited them is that AIDS stands as a catalyst for change in people's lives. It may well be "the disease of the week" on national TV, as well as headline-blaring fodder for newspapers. Yet the upheaval, even when it seems negative, works to raise the awareness of the persons involved. The positive news about AIDS and AIDS families now beginning to trickle into the media is a natural reaction against the negative barrage that has created hysteria for so long. Since AIDS seems to touch everyone you meet these days in some way or another, the confrontation process itself can be a healthy one. Family agonies can parallel global agonies. Family acceptance can parallel social changes.

For the shock of AIDS coming into your life can teach compassion as well as fear. And every reaction is a healing step, even though it doesn't seem so at the time. It is only when we hide our heads in the sand and refuse our feelings that we remain stuck and lost. By telling the truth, by speaking out in whatever way is possible for us, by reaching out to other families, we move from denial to acceptance. We then create a climate for the AIDS person to make his/her own choices, not to deny the facts about the disease but to move beyond that point to accept new possibilities for healing.

Healing is not exclusively the province of the AIDS patient. All of us touched by AIDS are healing ourselves too. Our capacity to love has no barriers. Our ability to heal ourselves in the midst of fear again has no barriers except those that we assign to ourselves.

When talking to AIDS families, I am reminded again and again of what Norman Cousins had to say about survival formulas. He said, in part:

> There is no single formula for human survival, but the approach to survival has two main elements:
>
> The first is that we ought never to minimize or underestimate the nature of the problems that confront us.
>
> The second is that we ought never to minimize or underestimate our ability to deal with them.

"Health is the result of relinquishing all
attempts to use the body lovelessly."
—A COURSE IN MIRACLES

7 ALTERNATIVE THERAPIES I

Interview with Steve Parrish, Pioneer Counselor Working with AIDS Patients

The following is a remarkable interview with Steve Parrish, certified rebirther and teacher of *A Course in Miracles.* Steve is a pioneer in that he is the first and to my knowledge the only rebirther whose practice now consists almost exclusively of AIDS patients and their families. My son Michael was his first AIDS client and the results in terms of Michael's healing of his relationships have been miraculous. Another son, Robert, and myself, have also experienced rebirthing sessions with Steve. Steve also assisted as a teacher during my own rebirthing training. In my opinion, Steve's presence in the room creates an atmosphere of peacefulness and trust. Soft-spoken and gentle, his quietness adds to his strength. By designing his entire practice around the principles of *A Course in Miracles,* he is able to reach out to his clients with unconditional love and assist them to discover their own capacity for love. His work with AIDS patients has real significance.

B.C.M.: Steve, what exactly *is* rebirthing? What can it do for the AIDS patient or other clients?

Steve: Rebirthing is a breathing exercise that releases emotions and old ideas about oneself that are literally stored physically in the body. This conscious, connected breathing, under the direction of an experienced rebirther, can regress the client back to the moment of birth and even beyond that, to emotional and physical sensations of being in the womb and then reexperiencing one's own birth. You see, right from the moment of birth or shortly afterward, I believe that most of us made most of our major decisions about life. At that time of intense vulnerability, pain, and shock, we decided, "I'm not alone. Life hurts. I'm not loved. I'm not wanted. I'm not big enough or strong enough or good enough." For most of us our early childhood experiences corroborated these initial impressions and literally built these emotional ideas into our body and mind where they became entrenched belief systems. Through these beliefs, held at an unconscious level, we viewed the world. Most of us are still operating from these old beliefs. Rebirthing seeks to provide a safe, loving place where we can experience these sensations, clear them out of the body and mind, so that our true self can emerge and can be all that we were meant to be.

B.C.M.: I understand, from technical writings about the rebirthing process, that it can literally change the limbic system, so that the person thinks and feels and behaves differently. There have been some studies on its ability to integrate the left brain and the right brain into a more unified whole.*

Steve: I am not familiar with those studies. I *do* know that rebirthing changes your stream of consciousness so that you approach life, including work, relationships, and indeed ev-

---

*"An Introduction to Rebirthing For Health Professionals," Eve Jones, Ph.D., from *Celebration of Breath*, Sondra Ray, Celestial Arts, Berkeley, Ca., 1983.

erything in the mundane world, with increased clarity and simplicity and, for most of us, in a more loving and responsible way. But rebirthing doesn't change who you essentially are; it just removes the blocks to love's awareness, removes the armor and the heaviness and distrust most people carry around with them for a lifetime. It brings the unconscious up to be observed, dealt with, and released safely, so that the client can then operate from a conscious level and make conscious choices about his or her life or death. Rebirthing doesn't change who you are; it just makes you more aware of who you are. You don't get to hide from yourself anymore.

B.C.M.: How can rebirthing help the AIDS patient to heal himself?

Steve: The AIDS patient has two choices. He can go the straight medical route, which so far has resulted in death, or he can choose alternative routes, which include rebirthing. At least with an alternative route the person has more choices about his own living or dying. He can choose to die gracefully, with dignity, after healing his relationships, which is a common theme among AIDS patients—"I want to heal all my relationships before I die." Since rebirthing is all about healing relationships with your parents, with yourself, with your relationship to God, then it is an effective route for the AIDS person to take. Or he can choose to live and do that through healing his past and healing his relationships.

B.C.M.: What about the AIDS person's fear of dying, of the gradual deterioration and mutilation of the body? Isn't that the major issue for the AIDS person to be concerned with?

Steve: Strangely enough, fear of dying is one of the *least* important issues for the AIDS clients who come to me. *The Course in Miracles* teaches that "I am not my body. I am free, I am as God created me." While the client and I address and assess *all* the major negatives that may have led the person to this disease, by the time I get the AIDS client, his major focus, again, is on healing his relationships, *all* his relationships, clearing up his act, so to speak. My clients are more interested in the quality of life they have left than the actual number of years involved. Strangely enough, my AIDS patients tell me that their lives are happier than they have ever been. They are more in touch with their feelings; they are more aware of love in all its forms. They do not fear death; they're committed to making their lives as meaningful as possible.

B.C.M.: This picture contrasts so sharply from the general public's view of AIDS patients, as fear-wracked, loathsome lepers waiting to die in agony, alone.

Steve: Well, I think timing is important here. Many AIDS patients, when they receive the current "death sentence" from their doctors, go home and shut themselves up in their rooms and wait to die. They shut out everyone and everything. They are then literally AIDS "victims," not persons who have a disease called AIDS. The disease could be cancer; it could be any one of a series of medical pronouncements. The person is going to use that medical vehicle to exit the planet. They are in such despair and rage that they can't conceive of *any* alternative. I'm lucky in that usually the people who seek me out, while initially still frightened and in despair, have chosen *not* to give up, have chosen to do what they can do to make their lives mean something, no matter how long that life may be. And as I said, the major issues for my clients revolve around healing relationships, especially parental relationships, and a major part of the work consists of releasing negative emotional blocks that stand in the way of that forgiveness.

B.C.M.: The goal of most psychotherapy seems to be the same: that of clearing up old patterns, especially involving childhood and parents. How does rebirthing, and specifically your practice, Steve, differ from traditional psychotherapy?

Steve: Rebirthing deals in *emotional therapy*, not mental therapy. The difference is that in traditional psychotherapy you try to figure it out. In rebirthing you *feel it out*. In rebirthing, the client is in an alpha state, sort of like self-hypnosis, and we can then use all kinds of self-help, therapeutic techniques to assist the client with "experiencing it out," reexperiencing the emotions and moving the energy out, rather than just realizing on a mental level that this is the way I am because my parents didn't love me, which is an untrue statement in itself, because it's not what really happened to the child that's important. It's the conclusions he drew about all these events that happened to him that's important. We want to go beyond the thinking portion of the mind and literally let go of the original emotion that created the thought pattern.

B.C.M.: Can you give me a specific example of how that works?

Steve: Yes. I remember one young man with AIDS I worked with for several sessions. Then, during one session, he became very agitated with the memory of having been seriously burned as a child of four or five. His dad had started a fire—I think it was to burn off some weeds—and my client had gone back later and imitated his dad starting a fire with matches and oil-soaked rags and had burned himself severely. During the course of the rebirthing, he literally reexperienced that fire at an emotional level and released the shock and trauma of that event. At that point I asked him to do some inner-child work.

B.C.M.: Inner-child work? Could you explain that?

Steve: Well, in this instance I had the young man go back to the original scene of his father starting the fire, and I had the young man go through a process in which he had an inner dialogue with his dad and in which he literally recreated the scene, so that his dad was explaining safety rules of fire and showing him how to start a fire and generally taking care of the young man so that the original fire experience became a pleasant one instead of a traumatic one. At the end of the process the young man hugged his dad in memory and thanked him for being there. The entire experience was a healing one for my client.

B.C.M.: So in inner-child work the client goes back in time and erases the past and recreates it the way he wants it?

Steve: Yes, but that's only a part of many ways in which the original rebirthing experiences can be expanded to help the client heal his past. I sometimes use mirror work, in which the client talks to the person, often dead, with whom he has had significant misunderstandings. This comes after a great deal of anger and sadness has been expressed physically by the patient through rebirthing breathing. I use a variety of ways in which to assist the client in moving the negative energy out of his body in safe ways. The inner-child part comes later in the session as integrative work, which is what healing is all about, integrating mind, body, and emotions.

B.C.M.: I have used inner-child work myself and have found it very effective. Why do you think it works?

Steve: In inner-child work you have the opportunity of going back to the past and reinterpreting the past, an opportunity we don't often get. You see, the inner child is magical. It's that part of ourselves that feels it can do anything. Inner-child work helps the mind to accept the new reality and puts the feeling child in charge of changing those emotions. It's a powerful, loving technique. Inner-child energy creates a shift within in order to change *current adult energy*.

B.C.M.: You also use inner-guide work, don't you?

Steve: Yes, I do. Often, near the end of a rebirthing session, I introduce the client to his own inner guide. He does this by going to a place within his heart center where he can allow the mind to be quiet and just listen. When the person contacts his inner guide, he can ask it what he needs to know next, and then just listen for guidance. He can use this inner guide in all aspects of his healing, not just during a rebirthing session. He can turn to his quiet place in his heart whenever he wants to, for guidance and strength.

B.C.M.: I also understand you use all kinds of spoken and written affirmations to help the client move past his present condition into new health.

Steve: I use whatever seems to work intuitively for the client. I am not a healer. I am not a rescuer. What I feel I am is a loving channel providing a safe space for the client to be healed. By turning over each and every rebirth to the Holy Spirit, as taught by *A Course in Miracles,* I can just get myself out of the way and let the healing take place. Every rebirth is unique and different. Every rebirth is only as effective as the space of love going into the process between rebirther and rebirthee. Success of the rebirth depends on both parties' willingness to surrender to the moment. So as a rebirther I am just here to assist the client in making conscious choices about his life.

B.C.M.: I know you tailor the sessions to the individual. How many sessions does the AIDS person usually require, how long are the sessions, and how are the AIDS client's sessions different from your regular sessions?

Steve: In general the AIDS patient, at the beginning, is more physically limited, so I have to tailor the sessions to what the AIDS person can handle at any given time. Generally rebirths last about one and a half hours, but with my AIDS clients we sometimes go for as long as three or four hours for total therapeutic time, although obviously not all that time is spent in the actual rebirth but in related integrative work. In theory, the client and I can go to the instant that predisposed the self to the AIDS, but in practice AIDS can be a conglomeration of past decisions about the client's life, AIDS being only an outer manifestation of what is going on with the person inside. Once we begin working with this matrix of the emotional past, we can, in later rebirths, go to the child within, find out the child's needs, and then give the child's needs to him in the form of intensive inner-child work.

B.C.M.: Is the AIDS person any different from your regular clients?

Steve: Every client is different. Every session is different. Generally, though, the rebirths with AIDS patients are much more intense than non-AIDS patients' rebirths. The AIDS client has already shifted his time frame in an interesting fashion. There's less drama involved with AIDS patients.

B.C.M.: Less drama? I thought there would be more.

Steve: In rebirthing, I define drama as the draping on top of real feelings. Drama is generally the imitation of feelings, not the real feelings themselves. AIDS patients deal more with their direct feelings. (After all, they've got nothing to lose!) They are generally more in touch with their real feelings, not necessarily consciously at first, but still, their real feelings are closer to the surface, easier to work with. They can work directly with their anger. Since anger breaks down the immune system, the emotional release of tons of anger during rebirthing is extremely valuable. A major component of rebirthing aims at removing stress from the body so that the body can heal itself. My AIDS clients can get past the drama into the trauma. Just as every rebirth is different, so the actual sessions needed are different. Usually clients go through a series of ten sessions, more if they want to or feel they need to. It all depends on the individual and the level of clearing desired. I know you've been through so many rebirths, you've lost count. So have I. Again, the person himself is the judge. Blocks concerning time, energy, or money also have to be worked out, although I never turn anyone away for lack of funds. It all depends on the person's commitment to his total healing. There's no pressure put on anybody. I don't go to the patient's home and drag him out and say, "You need to be rebirthed" or, "You need more healing. Come with me." People make their own choices daily. I'm just one way, one choice they have.

B.C.M.: I know the value of your work and the integrity of your commitment. Do you have anything else to add in conclusion?

Steve: Just this. We are all here to serve in love and to heal the planet. I simply assist people in uncovering the love within themselves. They can find their own way.

"I can elect to change all thoughts that hurt."

—A COURSE IN MIRACLES

8 ALTERNATIVE THERAPIES II

The "Love Your Self—Heal Your Body" Experience; The Hundredth Heart

The night I finally visited the "Love Your Self—Heal Your Body" Wednesday night group for gay men, mostly AIDS persons, facilitated by Louise Hay and Gisela Miller, I was weary almost to tears with exhaustion over the whole AIDS crisis. It seemed that I breathed, ate, slept, worked, counseled, and wrote, all under a huge umbrella called AIDS.

I had attended Louise Hay's Thursday night group several times, which was for everyone, not just for AIDS/gay people, and had gone away often with a positive feeling at the simple, loving support-group atmosphere that was familiar to me because of my own years of work in metaphysics, gone away calmed and nourished by the people who came to the group. I knew the entire staff at the "Love Your Self— Heal Your Body" Center, including the facilitators, Louise, Gisela and Jon Miller, and Linda Tilghman, and had found them to be dedicated, supportive workers who genuinely wanted to help others.

The Thursday night group was like a soothing tea in a nervous world, like a pep pill that encouraged me to go home singing the simple, sincere songs of affirmation we opened and closed the evening with. The group was held in a homelike atmosphere, in Louise's living room, and was a combination of singing, meditation, affirmative processes, a discussion, and sharing of insights by the group, followed by a healing circle that sent loving energy to the persons that night who seemed, in Louise's estimation, to need it most. Often people came to both the Wednesday and Thursday night groups; there was a lot of overlap, and many of the faces were familiar to me, most of them, (like me), involved in the AIDS phenomenon. The staff were always there, to help us give comfort to ourselves and to help us to learn to love ourselves more, which is a basic tenet of the "Love Your Self—Heal Your Body" organization. In that intimate, homelike atmosphere, where we hugged each other and hugged the teddy bears and the Hug-a-Planet stuffed balls in childlike consolation, where we wished, not on stars but on golden hearts; wished like this:

"May my heart open to others."

"I want to love unconditionally."

"I accept my magnificence now."

We were able to touch one another and to become, for a couple of hours at least, friends instead of strangers, as we let ourselves reach out to others as a part of a comforting group. Yet I had resisted the Wednesday night group for a long time. It was held an hour's drive away, in a large rented hall that also served as a gymnasium, and consisted of people with AIDS or ARC, plus a sprinkling of doctors, psychotherapists, nurses, and occasionally a family member. How overwhelming to walk into a group like that and be confronted all over again, not only with any remaining residue of fear concerning Michael's illness but also with my own ability or inability to handle whatever happened, life or death, in Michael's life. I remembered the last gay support group I had visited, and the climate of anger and fear that reigned, the barely veiled hostility at "straight" family members, the bravado, the exaggerated "camping." It had felt like an arena of despair, wherein I was expected to have total understanding for others, with no one being there for me. I felt then, as I felt now, as I walked into the Wednesday night group, that I was a stranger in a strange land. I felt that no matter how I directed my heart to love and accept others, no matter how I directed my mind to erase old cultural conditioning tapes, no matter how I directed my body to breathe and to relax, that I—not them—*I* was lacking in some fundamental way, that my courage, my caring, my very self was as alien to most of the audience as they were to me. I had accepted alternative life-styles within my family. I had accepted my children's gay friends. I had accepted my own gay friends, teachers, health professionals. And yet, and yet. Michael, dear Michael, child of my heart, this is so hard for me. This is a strange world for me. I've been a long time thinking in a certain way, and learning to love unconditionally isn't mastered overnight, no matter the willingness.

I was the only mother there. Oh, there was a woman therapist who worked with Carl Simonton's life-healing groups for cancer patients; there was a young woman with AIDS who had flown across the country to go through the "Love Your Self—Heal Your Body" intensive workshop; there were a couple of nurses. There was a male doctor who worked with AIDS patients and a man taking notes for healing tapes. There was also a camera crew because that night was one of two nights of videotaping for a documentary to be done on this group that would then be sent to other AIDS centers across the country. The familiar faces from the center were there, including my youngest son, Bob, who worked there and his friend, Steve, who had helped Michael so much and was an integral part of our family now. Louise Hay and Gisela Miller were there to facilitate the group.

And there were 250 or more gay men, who either had AIDS or ARC or had recovered from AIDS or ARC, and their newcomer friends who had come out of their own curiosity and fears about the disease, or who were in a relationship with other young men with AIDS or ARC.

Those who did not want to be on camera were on one side of the room, out of camera range, thus allowing for their fears at losing their jobs or their families to be allayed until they felt safe about speaking out publicly. The rest of us, those who lived and worked with the specter of AIDS daily, and those who had already "come out" about their sexual orientation and/or AIDS illness, were within camera range, on the hard floor or other equally hard chairs. For three hours we spoke about ourselves and about early patterns of illness, about childhood decisions, about both our fears and our triumphs.

Two nights earlier the landmark TV movie *An Early Frost*, the first movie to deal with the effects of AIDS upon a family, had aired. I believe that everyone in the room had been affected in one way or another by that movie, even those who said they had avoided watching it because of their own fears and because of previous overkill by the media in a fear-producing way. Some, like me, were exhausted by the whole AIDS situation, wanted to run and hide and get away from the mass hysteria and doom-filled prophecies they were encountering daily. For we were in the largest epidemic concentration of AIDS-involved persons in the country, where frenetic activity combined with fast-lane life-styles to produce a frantic, fear-filled atmosphere, where your friends, as one young man put it graphically, "died before your very eyes."

My son Bob spoke briefly and eloquently about sharing the TV movie experience with "his mom," and how much that had meant to him. I had not intended to say anything, but when I was called upon to share my feelings, I was able to affirm, from a deep place within my heart where I knew the words to be true, of the healing experience that Michael's illness had brought to the family. I don't remember exactly what I said. I talked about the need for healing relationships, especially family relationships. I talked about the gift that Michael's illness had brought to each of us in the family, as we learned to lay the past aside and to reach out to one another in love and acceptance, no matter what the situation, no matter what the consequences of the AIDS crisis in our lives. I spoke of family determination to use this experience as a healing one and to reach out and share the truth with others, each in our individual ways. And I talked about the "healing heart," because my initial reaction when I had walked into the room had dissipated, and the sore, frightened, overwhelmed heart within me now felt alive and well and, of its own accord, expanded itself out into the room.

There was a lot of expansion that night. There must have been at least a hundred other people who spoke out. Their stories run throughout this book and are a part of the fabric of healing that we felt in the room that night. The theme was that we are all healers of our own lives. We were all there to create the space and the safety to allow ourselves to reach our own insights and to begin to heal ourselves from within. Not a new concept surely, but one shared by many in the healing profession.

Three events stood out with clarity for me that evening. (To reproduce the whole evening would surely take another book).

One such insight came when Gisela spoke of the hundredth heart. Some of us had heard of the Hundredth Monkey Theory, (from Ken Keyes's book of the same name). This theory stated that when a civilization has gone as far as it can go and can see no way of expanding or going further, then the hundredth monkey somehow leaps across the barriers of space, like animals or birds who migrate in some inexplicable way to another shore, and that hundredth monkey is the one who makes the leap into the new, and from that act civilization expands, and we go on in an evolutionary journey that may involve many more leaps into the unknown by the hundredth monkey.

Gisela told the group, "The hundredth monkey is a phenomenon which we are seeing now, in which concepts and behavior changes leap across the world, transmitted as if on wires. And our work, in which people meet for the specific purpose of learning to love self and others; this, too, is springing up all over the world. But we are not dealing with a monkey. We are dealing with the heart. And the hundredth heart is a global affair."

For us to think of ourselves as "the hundredth heart" is surely more life-enhancing than to think of ourselves as family "victims" of this "incurable" disease. I looked around at the faces of the young men at the meeting, some still holding their stuffed toys or their "Hug-a-Planet" for comfort, and I saw the open, naked faces and the yearning within each of them to be a part of healing, instead of a part of disease.

As one young therapist from San Diego who works with *A Course in Miracles* put it, "The *Course* states that all illness comes from a lack of forgiveness. Surely if we learn anything from this horrible disease, it is that we must begin to forgive ourselves and others in order to be healed within, in order to make a difference in the world."

All was not sweetness and light. One young man told laughingly, but with a distinct tinge of bitterness in his voice, how he was diagnosed with AIDS about three years ago and told to go home and die. He realized that up to that point in his life he had depended on a doctor to tell him whether he was well or ill and had given all the power for his well-being over to an outside authority. He determined at that point to take his life into his own hands and began a program of diet, nutrition, exercise, therapy, any and all healing avenues; again, not taking other healing authorities as verbatim but finding his way with the help of various alternative sources. Three years later, the picture of health (and he was indeed a handsome, healthy-looking, glowing young man as he talked), he went back to his doctor to show him the "new man." His doctor then told him that all the initial tests and initial symptoms of the disease must have been wrong, there was no other explanation possible, and that the young man obviously never had had AIDS!

A wonderful doctor who works with AIDS patients responded. Dr. Robert Brooks, whose contribution appears in Chapter IV, "The Medical Aspects of AIDS," laughingly concurred that despite heroic measures by many concerned and compassionate doctors working with AIDS patients, many are as baffled as the rest of us out here because, as of this date, we don't know what heals or what doesn't heal. We only know about an epidemic that is so far supposedly incurable. We are not in opposite camps, battling each other over AIDS and its treatment. We are all working in our own way for health.

Dr. Brooks suggested that those of us that night *not* accept death sentences as infallible, *not* give the power of our own life or death into the hands of some outside authority but to recognize that the AIDS medical facts do leave doctors in the dark so far. Each person there could certainly take all precautions necessary against spreading the disease while taking pronouncements of doom with a grain of salt. He suggested that we use doctors and medical facts and laboratory findings as scientific testing agents as to the presence of Kaposi's sarcoma, T-cell deficiency, etc., but from that point onward, make our own choices about what to do about the information, and make our own choices about how to go about healing our lives.

There are as yet no firm statistics on living AIDS patients. The media continually insists that no one survives

AIDS. Yet all but one of the young people interviewed for this book are still living in apparent good health past all medical expectations. Each of them has one thing in common: an intense desire to live. None of them know when they are going to die, just as you or I do not know when we will die. For now they are all committed to life, no matter what outside health professionals may say.

Like Norman Cousins in *Anatomy of an Illness*, they use faith, hope, love, laughter, optimism, and vitamins (including megadoses of Vitamin C and homeopathic remedies). The *means* used are *not* what the AIDS person gives power to. Means, after all, are just that, specific helps in repairing the physical body to a specific conclusion. Yet none of these young men and one woman have blindly accepted radiation or chemotherapy (more poisons to kill the poisons). Instead those I know still living with the AIDS virus have refused, for the most part, the standard medical route, or if they did take the standard medical route, have assisted the healing process themselves by using alternative methods to increase their lifespans. They have, in all cases that I knew of, taken responsibility for their inner regeneration through holistic avenues.

This is not as radical as it may sound. Again and again doctors say that nature cures the patient, not doctors, that the patient's will to live, followed by constructive action to implement that will (including mind/body aids) is the factor that sways the balance between accepting death and choosing to fight for life. Some do not win that fight. But for the young men in the room that night, a chance was offered. The evidence presented by those still living was that life could be an alternative to the almost certain AIDS death they had expected.

"I refuse to roll over and play dead," commented one.

"I have already walked through the valley of the shadow," said another, "and God is with me."

For those with AIDS who were still reeling with shock at their diagnosis, the self-confidence, candor, and obvious well-being of the young men speaking out offered more than just hope.

"If you can do it, I can do it," said one young man who had been diagnosed with Kaposi's sarcoma only three days earlier.

Another event that impressed itself upon my heart occurred after the group had broken up for the evening. A vibrant, healthy-looking young man in a wildly striped pink-and-white shirt that reminded me of the candy striper uniforms worn by hospital volunteers (indeed, he had reminded me of a cheerful hospital volunteer all evening) came over to me to tell me how much my "sharing" had meant to him. Earlier I had learned that he had AIDS in the form of Kaposi's sarcoma, with lesions in his mouth that now seemed to be healing.

"I'm Richard, from Houston," he announced, "And I just want to shake your hand."

I put my arms around him instead and gave him a heartfelt hug.

He had tears in his eyes. "Some people aren't willing to do that," he said wistfully. "So I always offer them a chance to shake my hand instead. At least that's some contact. I miss my mom," he continued. "We hardly ever get any moms here."

So I hugged him again, tears in my eyes as well.

"Hey, guys," he said, "we don't need the Hug-a-Planet anymore. We've got a Hug-a-Mom instead." And he then and there nominated me to be his Hug-a-Mom and began lining up other of his friends for hugs. Well, how can you refuse a candy striper? So now I am an official Hug-a-Mom.

I want to give full credit to *all* who are working in loving, inspiring ways to help AIDS patients and their families. For me these Wednesday and Thursday night evenings were a part of my own healing, and I returned to them often, not as a reporter or researcher, but as a mother whose son had AIDS.

And I am still working daily with my own healing heart, as well as being a part of the hundredth heart.

It was with this feeling that I approached my interviews with the staff of the "Love Your Self—Heal Your Body" Center. While I recognize that there are other inspiring groups all over the country now working with AIDS patients, working with other types of catastrophic illness and their effects, and/or working in holistic healing fields that stress the connection between the mind, the body, and the emotions in healing one's life, I also recognize that for Michael, Louise Hay's tape entitled "AIDS: A Positive Approach" was an important source of encouragement for my son and other AIDS patients. It was a key of value, one within which they found that they could indeed change their minds from a death sentence to a life sentence. From their exposure to the tape many AIDS patients have reported to me that they now utilize both conventional medical means and other holistic healing tools in conjunction with the Hay approach.

I chose to interview Gisela Miller of the "Love Your Self—Heal Your Body" Center, Louise's co-facilitator, whose credentials include certification as a minister in the Church of Religious Science, as well as many years working as a metaphysical counselor and seminar leader (Louise's credentials are similar), to share with me some of the healing techniques that are offered in the intensive, five-day workshops given periodically by the Center. It is certain that the love that flows from these healing helpers has touched the lives of thousands of AIDS patients, as well as countless others who attend the events at the Center. In addition, the ideas and techniques presented in this chapter can be used immediately for beneficial results by the reader.

B.C.M.: Gisela, when did the "Love Your Self—Heal Your Body" Center begin to counsel specifically with AIDS patients?

Gisela: We started in January 1985, with six men who had AIDS. This was a one-week residential program now called the intensive workshop. These AIDS patients lived with Louise in her home for one week while they cleared away the patterns that they discovered were at the root cause of their illness. We also included extensive bodywork, massage, etc., nutritional counseling, and private and group therapy that we consider spiritually based with sound psychological principles. Then the first Wednesday night group for gay men/people with AIDS started in March 1985. We already had a Thursday night group for the general public.

B.C.M.: Describe what goes on in the intensive workshop.

Gisela: We treat the whole person, body, mind, and spirit. This is an immersion workshop. People just dive in for five days. We call in a staff of experts to help us, and the intensive includes everything mentioned in the first residential program, plus a complete astrological workup (to see where the person is in terms of developing future potential and soul growth). We also do neuro-linguistic programming, taught by my husband, Jon Miller, who's the Executive Director of the Center.

I want to emphasize that the intensive is tailored for each individual, not just AIDS patients. Right now we're getting mostly AIDS clients, because it's such an urgent, life-threatening disease. People come to us from all over the country, many with severe health problems that do not include AIDS.

B.C.M.: I'm curious about the type of person that would come from across the country to really face themselves. What's the common denominator with AIDS patients?

Gisela: They come in as very intense, driven individuals without a lot of self-love or self-appreciation. After the intensive they usually understand that they have a choice to live or die and by then they have dissolved many of the old resentments that have kept them from loving the self. The common denominator we see is guilt, especially sexual guilt. In addition, these clients are usually estranged from their parents, but this is not limited to just family members. They are usually estranged from everyone around them. When they come to us, they are already committed to healing themselves. They have made the choice consciously. And the first thing they have to do is give up their "victim" act. You *cannot* heal yourself and still operate in the world as a "victim," the old they-did-it-to-me mentality.

B.C.M.: So it's not all sweetness and light and positive thinking in the intensive, Gisela?

Gisela: Not at all. In group work we get down to the negatives that run a person's life. We work at the cell level to reprogram the personal belief system. We use everything we know to help the person to break through self-imposed barriers and see himself in a different light.

B.C.M.: How could five days, in all honesty, make such a difference in a person's life that he or she could reverse what some people call a death sentence?

Gisela: When clients go back out into the world, they are provided with so many tools to keep them focused and on track. For example, after learning NLP, they can develop self-programming helps called "anchors" to recall their real strength and power. Also, we do a lot of mirror work, and students are encouraged to do this technique each day at home. This is a daily process of forgiving self and others. Students are given lots of phone numbers to call for support, and we have a phone counseling line here at the Center.

Those who live in this area usually continue in private counseling and in the Wednesday or Thursday night groups. There are also regular two-day seminars for all to attend. In these two-day seminars we can present some of the same information we use in the intensive, although obviously we use different techniques when dealing with 300 or 400 people at a time, rather than in a small group setting. But we can present six or eight major life-changing exercises within the setting, and then people take what they can use and go on from there. The ultimate outcome for all the work we do here is that people leave with a greater sense of love and understanding for themselves.

B.C.M.: Tell me about a specific process of healing that the client and the reader can do for themselves.

Gisela: I believe that mirror work is the most powerful tool that the client can use to work with all parts of the emerging self, the client's child, the intellect of that child within, and the parental intellect as well. We're talking about one person here, not just the personality we present to the outside world. You have to know yourself before you can heal yourself.

Mirror Work Technique

Sit down and take some time to look into a mirror and begin to know the person within you. (If you stand, you will be tempted to run away.) A full-length mirror is best, but use whatever you have at hand.

Look deep within your own eyes. Bring forth the little child that lives within you. Introduce yourself to that child. Talk to that little girl or boy in the mirror. Get to know that person. Tell the child in the mirror how much you love it. Forgive the child within for any mistakes ever made. Let the little child within talk to you and then forgive you (the adult self) for not taking better care of it. Whisper a special secret in that little child's ear: something (you will know what it is) that the child of you has always wanted to hear from you.

Now reach out in your imagination and let the big child of you hold the little child of you until the little child is dissolved into the center of your chest at the heart level. Visualize picking up and holding that beautiful, special child within you. You are creating a reunion of the selves. You are one with your own child self. Pledge to yourself that from this moment on you will always love and take care of that child within you.

By doing this mirror-work exercise and any other spontaneous mirror-work processes that may come to you as you work at forgiving the self daily, you can learn to renegotiate new agreements with yourself. According to Gisela, mirror-work processes put the person in charge or his or her own belief systems. Of course, the client is already using many other visualizations to help heal the self, as well as specific homework assignments, some written, some oral, to point the person toward inner healing.

B.C.M.: What would you like to tell everyone about this work that all of you do at the Center?

Gisela: The work we do here is just a vehicle for getting several powerful methods of healing under one roof in a concentrated period of time so that the people involved learn how to move to the other side of major obstacles they are holding on to. These obstacles may be AIDS, or they may be work, relationships, money, etc. We teach the person to break through self-imposed barriers.

B.C.M.: What are your future plans for this work?

Gisela: To hold the space so that people can feel safe enough to heal themselves. We want to do everything within our power to let it be known that wellness is a natural state of living. We are continually expanding, creating new books, new tapes, a video, working all over the country in churches and halls, with thousands of people, to help people learn to heal themselves. Louise and I want to emphasize that we do not heal anyone. We do provide the space, time, energy, love, and tools that enable people to heal themselves within (whatever form that may take), or, at the least, help the person to recognize the nonhealing stumbling blocks that may have contributed to his current state of illness and, from that recognition, help the person to relearn, to rechoose new ways of living. And everyone—I mean everyone!—can do this.

Every time I go into the "Love Your Self—Heal Your Body" Center, I am amazed at the positive, dedicated people who use the basic processes discussed earlier within their work environment. I asked Bob Welsch to answer three questions about his work with AIDS persons.

B.C.M.: What do you think is the major problem AIDS patients and families face when healing themselves?

Bob Welsch: To stay on track with their healing; to be really clear that their diagnosis is like the balance on an account. It is the state of the body at a particular moment in time. If the person continues to affirm wellness, not illness, and has the support of the family in affirming wellness also, then that person is on the way to healing. The biggest problem is the negative media and the mass consciousness they project of the AIDS person being a "fatal victim." This attitude is damaging and only serves to promote the virus of fear.

B.C.M.: Bob, what is the most important contribution you make toward healing the planet through your work at the Center?

Bob Welsch: To teach only love. Also, I find that I must take my own responsibility in healing the planet. This was difficult for me at first. I continually choose to know that this is one of the reasons I'm here alive at this time, to help, through love.

B.C.M.: Bob, what's the one thing you would like to tell parents and friends of those with AIDS?"

Bob Welsch: Hug the person who has AIDS. Touch them, love them, show them you care. Also, I like to tell them that AIDS is here for them for a reason; that it may be an intense experience, and that there are many lessons to learn from this experience, whether we are the person or we are part of the family circle. We can all move through this experience individually and collectively and become better people because of it. All of us have the opportunity to look at new ways of being intimate with each other, showing our love for each other. This has nothing to do with sex or our sexual orientation. This is using love to heal past differences, past pains and hurts. Also, the AIDS experience is an opportunity to take one day at a time and just be in the moment, living where we are, and to rejoice in life together. And that's what *is* healing our lives! So even if we are physically separated by distance or death, there will be memories of joy and life to join us. Remember, *love heals*.

"It takes great learning to understand
that all things, events, encounters, and circumstances
are helpful."

—A COURSE IN MIRACLES

9

THERE'S A LOT MORE
HELP OUT THERE

Years ago I had boxes and boxes of personal stationery printed for me with the following message: "You deserve a miracle . . . so expect one today." I'm still using both the stationery and the message. This seems even more appropriate now as I connect with loving, caring groups of people who are working within their various belief systems to assist the AIDS person and the AIDS family toward healing and acceptance.

As AIDS becomes the number-one disease threat of the twentieth century, expected to assume plaguelike proportions that cut across gender, race, and class lines, there are hopeful beacons in the world. There are health professionals, various psychological counselors, and support groups of every kind. As new information about the mind/body connection reaches public awareness, there will be even more. In addition to the therapeutic help that Michael received from Steve Parrish, inner-child worker/rebirther, and the "Love Your Self—Heal Your Body" work with AIDS persons, there are several more facilities that I am aware of that assist the AIDS person and his family to move through crisis.

One such group is called, appropriately, "Expect a Miracle." It is based in San Francisco and is a nonprofit organization run by James C. Baker, who has an M.S. in Holistic Studies, and his partner, Jeffrey Boggs. In addition, "Expect a Miracle" uses a number of specially trained group helpers, (Michael was one of them), and utilizes therapeutic professionals from the community to present informative lectures in such fields as acupuncture, rebirthing therapy, kundalini yoga, nursing care, meditation techniques, and other alternative therapies.

"Expect a Miracle" is the toughest support group for AIDS persons that I have encountered, with a list of wide-ranging therapeutic techniques that force the participants to identify their basic life themes, take total and complete responsibility for everything they have created in their lives, including the disease AIDS, and then change their behavior patterns (not just their old thoughts), take complete and total responsibility for either living or dying, and commit themselves to an intensive, time-consuming, energy-restructuring program. According to Michael, who went through their program, and assisted newcomers in the program, "Expect a Miracle" uses such elements as psychodrama, a written autobiography, complete with family pictures of significant events in the person's life, intense self-questioning processes, goal-setting, integrity checklists with present and future timeline goals, and a host of eclectic therapeutic techniques.

I visited one "Expect a Miracle" workshop and was impressed at the sheer amount of work the participants had done, their honesty and clarity, and their group processes. "Expect a Miracle" can be an overwhelming commitment to make in one's life. The assignments, especially the written ones, require hours of work daily, and the components of the change process, an actual review and restructuring of the AIDS person's life, can bring up fearful feelings. The change process has often been compared to taking the lid off a volcano.

There is also an urgent quality to the "Expect a Miracle" processes. It's as if the participants have got to hurry up and do it; i.e., change their lives fast while they still have lives to change. The participants are required—not urged but *required*—to discover and uncover exactly what their relationships with others (especially family members) are all about, and then assisted in clearing up these relationships and in taking total responsibility for everything that is happening in their lives, especially their illness. "Expect a Miracle" now includes people who do not have AIDS or ARC but nevertheless want a tough transformational program. The focus remains the same. Face yourself. Face your past. Face your present. Put it all together. Process it out. Move forward with definite, planned, purposeful goals for your future. Then go out and help others to do the same. Needless to say, with such a tough program, many of the initial participants drop out when self-discovery brings to light their own participation in the tragedies of their lives, including the "payoffs" of their own victimization.

The facilitators of "Expect a Miracle" are now moving past the experimental stage and intend to work in gentler ways, more in keeping with the ideas expressed in *A Course in Miracles*, whose tenets are also an integral part of their individual focus. They are now leading advanced workshops, as well as the initial cram course in confrontation.

"Expect a Miracle," as well as all the other helping programs mentioned in this book, are listed in the bibliography, should anyone want to contact them personally.

I wasn't able to visit every AIDS project, every AIDS support group, the SHANTI projects (which work with the dying), or every organization working with AIDS patients and their families. I do want to mention two further groups of special interest to families whose loved one has been diagnosed with a usually fatal disease.

When another family had a bout with cancer several years ago, I immediately recommended *Getting Well Again*, by Simonton, Simonton, and Creighton. The Simontons' imagery techniques to assist cancer patients to heal themselves, while at the same time availing themselves of sound medical care, have now been expanded to include work with seriously ill patients with AIDS (recognizing that Kaposi's sarcoma, one of the manifestations of AIDS, is indeed a cancer), and other so-called fatal illnesses as well. They initially started in Fort Worth, Texas, ironically enough, just eight blocks from where I previously lived for so many years. I remember going past the tall white building with columns, which was located, providentially, right across the street from a major area hospital and cancer clinic and laboratory and wondering what went on there that helped so many people. Now, of course, there are Simonton clinics in other areas, including the Los Angeles area. Their work with the families, as well as the ill person, is effective, and I recommend them highly for anyone connected with the AIDS spectrum of illness or any terminal illness.

Another group that has gained worldwide attention in helping people deal with and, in some cases, healing catastrophic illness, is the Center for Attitudinal Healing, founded and directed by Dr. Gerald Jampolsky, and located in Tiburon, California. Through the application of *A Course in Miracles*, combined with the practice of unconditional love, Dr. Jampolsky's center has been able to make remarkable changes in the way people perceive themselves, others, and illness. In a previous book of mine I spoke of Gerald Jampolsky's work with *A Course in Miracles* within the context of the forgiveness principle. His books—*Love Is Letting Go of Fear, Teach Only Love, There is a Rainbow Behind Every Dark Cloud,* and *Saying Goodbye to Guilt*—are all favorites of mine that have helped me through dark days past, present, and I am sure, future.

I have a page from *Teach Only Love* taped to my refrigerator door. I read it every day. It helped me through my own illness as well as Michael's illness again and again when I became discouraged during the healing process. I would like to share it with you, with Dr. Jampolsky's permission.

According to Dr. Jampolsky, these are the seven principles of healing as explained in *The Course in Miracles*.

The Seven Principles

1. Health is inner peace. Therefore, healing is letting go of fear. To make changing the body our goal is to fail to recognize that our single goal is peace of mind.

2. The essence of our being is love. Love cannot be hindered by what is merely physical. Therefore we believe the mind has no limits; nothing is impossible; and all disease is potentially reversible. And because love is eternal, death need not be viewed fearfully.

3. Giving is receiving. When our attention is on giving and joining with others, fear is removed and we accept healing for ourselves.

4. All minds are joined. Therefore, all healing is self-healing. Our inner peace will of itself pass to others once we accept it for ourselves.

5. Now is the only time there is. Pain, grief, depression, guilt, and other forms of fear disappear when the mind is focused in loving peace on this instant.

6. Decisions are made by learning to listen to the preference for peace within us. There is no right or wrong behavior. The only meaningful choice is between fear and love.

7. Forgiveness is the way to true health and happiness. By not judging, we release the past and let go of our fears of the future. In so doing, we come to see that everyone is our teacher and that every circumstance is an opportunity for growth in happiness, peace, and love.

   Because of my own continuing involvement in working with the principles contained in *A Course in Miracles*, I would like to add that there are numerous groups all over the country who use these ideas as an integral part of their belief systems, whatever their religious preferences (or lack of).

   Principles of love, forgiveness, acceptance, and oneness with God are a part of my life and can be helpful in any situation requiring trust. Prayer, whatever form it takes as regards denomination, is to me, more than an alternative way of healing. It, too, is a part of my life. However, this book is not intended to proselytize for any one method of spiritual or psychological or medical help. Instead, a balanced review of specific alternative healing processes that were helpful in Michael's journey through illness and in my own involvement with his life-threatening disease, are presented in the hope that any or all of these suggestions may be just what is needed for you, as a parent or friend, at this point in your loved one's healing.

   In addition, I have been given helpful ideas that have worked for other AIDS persons. I offer any and all of these suggestions with a medical disclaimer. I am not a doctor, nor am I prescribing anything from acupuncture to the laying on of hands. I want to be especially emphatic when I talk about nutritional possibilities, even though I have seen improvement in AIDS conditions when the sound principles of nutrition, exercise, relaxation, and meditation techniques are followed along with the medical recommendations of the attending physician.

Some AIDS persons have used the following to help fortify their immune systems and to create a more favorable climate for detoxification of existing viruses: Immunplex (a standard-process homeopathic aid); large doses of Vitamin C; Spirulina (for its concentrated beta-carotene, thought to be a cancer fighter); and LaPacho tea (Pau'D'Arco tea), thought to help rid the body of parasites and fungal growths. In addition, Michael used various Chinese herbs for detoxification, taken only under the advice and care of his acupuncturist, Misha Cohen, as well as taking a host of homeopathic remedies while under the care of Dr. Lorraine Bonte, our family chiropractor, whose treatments helped Michael a great deal after his bout with fungal meningitis.

The emphasis here is on the patient taking responsibility for his health in conjunction with his attending physician's diagnosis. Until a cure is found for AIDS and all its opportunistic manifestations, anything and everything that can increase the well-being of the AIDS person and help each one to rebuild his body defenses can be utilized with optimistic results.

There is a lot more help out there! These suggestions are only a small part of what is becoming more available every day, as dedicated health-care professionals in many fields reach out to help the AIDS patient and the AIDS family. The trinity of mind, body, and spirit working together can ease each person's pain (whether physical or emotional) during the AIDS crisis and can help each of us to integrate holistic healing tools into the very fabric of our lives.

Practical, day-to-day advice is available too. At a recent

meeting of hospital personnel, mostly home health care and discharge planners, I was asked to contribute my thoughts about being a parent of someone who has AIDS. One of the areas of emphasis in my speech, beyond the obvious recommendations gleaned from the book in process, was a suggestion that the medical personnel concerned with the AIDS crisis understand and allow the AIDS person to explore any and all alternative processes that assisted in easing the patient and his family during the course of the illness. I was not arguing for alternative medicine as opposed to the medical model. I was not advocating that the patient walk away from health care and experiment solely on his own. What I did suggest was that the health personnel involved understand, encourage, and accept the person's responsibility of *choice*. As we find our way through the conflicting attitudes and recommendations concerning the care of AIDS, our belief systems can serve us well as we use every avenue— mind/body/spirit—as pathways to a total program of health care.

The other two speakers on the program, one a social worker from the AIDS Project, L.A., named Sally Jue, and the other a man named David Kessler, a male nurse who is the director of Progressive Nursing Services, a health-care company that takes care of bedridden AIDS patients, were valuable to me as they answered the practical questions of living and caring for a person with AIDS in a home setting. I also remember the concern and the obvious dedication of the hospital personnel who asked questions such as the following.

How great were the risks? What could we do to help AIDS patients be more comfortable without being paranoid ourselves? Did you indeed need masks and double gloves and double lab coats to approach an AIDS patient, as some doctors now did? Could you touch the person? Just how did one care for a severely ill person in the home without contracting the disease? These were not scare questions, but an honest concern for both the patient and the care-giver. None of these health professionals wanted to be like the ambulance attendants who refused to pick up AIDS patients or the funeral attendants who refused the bodies of AIDS patients. Neither did anyone want to be careless about spreading infection with a still relatively unknown disease.

I spoke candidly about Michael's visits to me, and my visits to him. He was a fanatic about cleanliness. I was not. You could not only eat off his floors; you could be assured that for Michael, cleanliness was not only next to godliness, it was an important indication to him that he had order in his life; that by living in a spotless environment, with everything in its place, he had control over his life in other ways. Yet, when he visited me and other family members, we fixed meals and washed dishes by hand; we took the laundry to the Washeteria. The floors and bathroom and kitchen were clean but not sterile, and most importantly, I hugged Michael a lot. So did the rest of his family. That nonjudgmental, accepting contact is vital, I believe, in the care of any person with a disease. No, I did not drink out of Michael's glass, eat off his plate, or use his towel or washcloth. Utensils were washed in very hot water, but a dishwasher would have been more sterile. Michael disposed of his own tissues after coughing and cleaned up the bathroom after himself. Both of us knew that casual contact does not spread AIDS. Neither of us wanted fear to be a part of our relationship. The most heartbreaking thing for an AIDS patient, I believe, is to be treated as an unclean, disease-carrying, walking time bomb.

In an interview with David Kessler, he reinforced and elaborated on the concerns generated in the meeting. David, an R.N., started Progressive Nursing Services when he discovered that there was no health care available for AIDS patients to be cared for at home. His logo states that respect, understanding, and quality care are what he and his staff strive to provide for the AIDS patients they treat. In my interview with David he stated emphatically that taking care of an AIDS patient is like taking care of any other sick person, that normal nursing procedures are followed to the letter. In his *Precautions for Health-Care Workers,* a pamphlet he has prepared for his nursing staff, he gives the following advice: Use gloves when handling body fluids (standard nursing procedure), and the rest of the time, as in giving a back rub or combing a patient's hair, forget about gloves and use as much soothing touch as possible when caring for the patient in day-to-day interactions. David feels that masks are not necessary and that normal procedures of cleanliness and disposal are sufficient when caring for an AIDS patient at home. He emphasized to me that he felt that an unknown diagnosis (such as what usually happens when patients first come into the hospital with something like tuberculosis or other diseases that then have to be verified by tests) is *more* risky for nurses than dealing with the known AIDS diagnosis.

"AIDS is a behavioral disease," David told me. "That means that you have to do something outside of day-to-day nursing care to contract it. It is extremely hard for health-care workers to get AIDS. In fact," he continued emphatically, "according to the *Journal of the AMA,* 'At this time all statistics of Health Care Workers with needle-stick injury (dealing with AIDS patients) are not at high risk.' " (Volume 254, Number 15, October 18, 1985.)

I asked David to tell me what he thought was the most important information he could share with the readers of this book.

"It's this," he stated. "There is no disease more isolated, more lonely, than AIDS. Therefore I believe that a parent's love is the most important factor in helping the AIDS patient. There is *nothing* more important than this! I repeat—*nothing!* This is the most devastating disease I know of, and

for a person to get well he must have that love." The AIDS
Project, L.A., also offers concrete, medically based advice
about caring for an AIDS patient in the home, whether the
patient is caring for himself with a little additional help or
being cared for by family, friends, or nursing personnel.

According to their publication entitled *Living With AIDS:
A Self-Care Manual*, anyone taking care of an AIDS patient
should not only use the normal precautions of washing hands
before and after touching a patient and the normal precautions of cleanliness regarding utensils, laundry, a clean house,
etc., but they also suggest wearing rubber gloves when
taking care of the intimate personal needs of a bedridden
patient, while cleaning the bathroom, and while disposing of
soiled items, syringes, etc.

The information contained in this manual is extremely
valuable for anyone who has AIDS or has a family member
with AIDS, and I recommend it without reservation. Since
the material is so extensive, the AIDS Project, L.A., sug-
gests that you study the entire manual and prefers that large
amounts of the manual not be excerpted at this time in other
publications. The importance of the information in this manual cannot be overlooked for anyone who has AIDS or is
connected in any way with someone who has AIDS. I strongly
urge a copy for everyone who reads this book and am
appreciative of the fine work by doctors and other health
professionals that went into the making of *Living With AIDS:
A Self-Care Manual*.

I am still learning about the help that exists for AIDS
patients and their families and friends. The quotation that
began this chapter tells it all: "It takes great learning to
understand that all things, events, encounters, and circumstances are helpful."

We are on the razor blade of choice as we move through
the various paths that offer healing and comfort during the
AIDS epidemic. And we must make our own choices as we

continue through the AIDS crisis. As more is learned about AIDS there will be even more choices available, even more concrete help for those of us who have someone we love who has AIDS.

10 BEYOND LIFE AND DEATH

Acceptance and Inner Peace

At one of the lowest points of Michael's illness, when I was not sure that he would live, when I was not sure if I could survive his illness or his possible death, I went to an early church service at Unity by the Sea, an area church. I went alone, just before Thanksgiving, and as I sat there quietly, not really meditating, because the storms of despair warred too strongly within me for that, but just sitting there, I asked, as I had so often, to be given the strength by God to get through this crisis. I believe that every person reading this book must have felt like I did at that moment. I imagine that each of you, all the mothers and fathers and brothers and sisters and grandparents and friends, must have asked again and again, not *what* to do about the situation of a loved one's tragic and usually fatal illness but simply *how*—how in the name of heaven do those of us watching a loved one's suffering, watching, in so many cases, a loved's one's death, get through it all? We are asking, in that moment, for ourselves, not them.

At that time Michael had developed a severe cold and cough from riding his motor scooter in the cold, soaking rain of a San Francisco autumn, home from support-group meet-ings where he helped other young men with AIDS. The dread word *pneumocystis* kept floating into my mind. I knew that a person with AIDS, no matter how well he seems to be recovering, is vulnerable to this form of pneumonia that is thought to be fatal at this time.

Michael had at this time survived the fungal meningitis. He had survived the Kaposi's sarcoma, although he still had lesions. He had survived a further operation in which lesions were cut out of his mouth so that he could breathe and eat. How much more could he take?

I valued Michael. I admired his courage, his determina-tion, his willingness to look within and change himself, his never-say-die attitude. I knew that Michael was using every ounce of faith he possessed to regenerate his own life. He was also using what strength he had to help others. He was a living, breathing miracle to those around him. He was not only determined to live but determined, as well, to have his life be a witness to others, an example that you *can* heal yourself, you *can* heal your relationships, you *can* start over, you *can* give your life to a higher purpose and a higher power.

Again and again Michael had said to me, "Mother, AIDS has awakened me. I am not concerned anymore with healing myself of AIDS. AIDS is not the issue. I am con-cerned only about healing my life and assisting others to heal theirs. My life is not about AIDS anymore. My life is about healing. My life is about reaching out in love."

And each time Michael said these words to me, I again and again spoke my own litany of prayer. "Michael, oh, Michael, child of my heart, don't die. You have so much to give."

Do any of us have any control over death? I remem-bered a woman who came to me for counseling. She worked daily with dying AIDS patients. The anger she felt far surmounted any other feelings she might have. In her zeal to help, she was battling against death. At the same time she was absolutely convinced that no one ever survived AIDS. She refused to listen to Michael's moving testimony of what he was doing in order to get well. She refused to consider any suggestions for help for herself in order to relieve the obvious unremitting stress she was under. This, although she had come obstensibly for help. She was battling death and yet, at the same time, convinced that she could not win. She railed against everyone from "do-gooders," as she called them, to doctors, to the media, to the general public. She was consumed with hatred and, at the same time, valiant in her efforts to help. I could not help but wonder how the recipients of her earnest crusade felt when she appeared at their bedside. Did her furious tirades against everyone from the government's indifference to the medical profession's ineptitude assist her in her volunteer work? Did anger alone keep her alive? If she let down her guard against the furious tide of death she was attempting to stem, would she be like the sorcerer's apprentice in *Fantasia*; would she simply go on exhausting herself trying to sweep out a flood that had already overwhelmed her? And yet she *was* helping, in her own way. She *did* care. And who was I to judge anyone else's way of dealing with death? For that is what she seemed to be doing, confronting death daily, and in so doing, confronting her own fears of death.

Isn't that what the doctors and nurses and social workers and psychiatrists did who worked with AIDS patients? Isn't that what most of us did when embroiled in a loved one's struggle with AIDS? Granted, we all met our fear of death in different ways. But meet death we did, and working through the anger and the fear was—*is*!—a part of that process of confrontation.

I remember an older man sitting on my couch in despair. His eyes and nose dripped rivulets as he told of the desperation he faced, the failures in his life, his son's AIDS illness that he didn't believe, couldn't believe, would be healed. Beyond his helplessness and hopelessness there was a great deal of anger that he refused to face. There was anger at himself for not being a better parent (ah, how familiar to all of us *that* one!), anger at the world for treating him so badly (in his estimation), and, with all his frightened tears, an enormous reservoir of self-pity. He felt that God (in whom he had never believed) had, nonetheless, *done* this to him. As I listened to him and did my best to comfort him, I realized that he had a laundry list of grievances against God. This laundry list included everything everyone had ever *done* to him, coupled with a desperation that he could no longer manipulate outer events, circumstances, or people to his will. I knew of this man's past patterns, both the love he had for his children and the mistakes he had made. I did not like this man. And yet he was so human! He, like everyone I had met in the course of my journey through the AIDS phenomenon, was deserving of time, of attention, of respect.

For we all meet the threat of death in different ways. There is no wrong or right way. I, too, had felt the anger and the self-pity, just as he had. I, too, like Job, had made out my list of grievances against the Almighty. I had struggled and screamed in my personal drama. Yet all I could think of as I listened to this man was: "This is not about death. This is about life and how each of us will live it from this point on."

At another crisis point in my life, I went for a walk along the marina. On one side was the calm placidity of the bay where sailboats floated on the still waters. On the other side was the full force of the Pacific Ocean, wave after wave lashing upon the rocks and the shoreline, wave after wave of the forces of nature coming, ever coming, until it seemed as if no one person could ever stand against that mighty, impersonal, implacable tide but would instead be swept away, overwhelmed, defeated, by the same God who made the tides, who made the ocean, who made Michael, who made me. I had no answers for myself at that time, no comforting platitudes to help me in my despair. I simply stood there and let a tidal wave of feelings engulf me as if I were, in fact, within the sea.

Like countless others before me, I begged God to save my son, begged God, that mighty, impersonal, implacable force, to listen to me, to hear my plea, to save me as well. I did not know how to go on. I did not know what to do next. How could I help Michael when I had no resources left within me? And how could I ever have the temerity to reach out to others, to put my feelings on paper and trust that they would be an opening for others to find their way through despair and into a place of acceptance and love?

I remember screaming inside myself, "I can't do it. I can't save Michael with my love. I can't write the book or give speeches or counsel with other parents. I don't know how. I don't know how to go on."

And the ocean just kept right on coming, roaring its way into my heart. The ocean didn't care. Neither, it seemed, did God, that mighty, implacable force that I could not stand against. Oh, of course, I also had a personal God, the loving, caring, nourishing God within me that helped me to be the best human being I knew how to be, the God that forgave my mistakes, that helped me to dry my tears, that helped me to get up in the morning and go on. That God seemed puny and ineffectual at this point: no match for the mighty forces that threatened Michael's life and, it seemed at that moment, my life as well. What did it matter, after all, if one more person lived or died, if one more mother loved or lived, if one more book got written, if one more hand reached out to another?

What did it matter, after all, if we loved one another?

For my love was not enough to save Michael from death, just as my love had not been enough to keep anyone in my life from death, not my daddy, not my grandmother, not my grandson. My love was not enough to keep people alive, or marriage alive, or love alive. And all my struggles to the contrary were just that—struggle. For Michael would choose, at some level of his being, to live or to die. Or God would choose the time for him. Or maybe it would be a combination of both, the human will and the Divine Will, so that Michael would walk through the door into another dimension, into another life, with his hand in God's hand, being led gently forward.

I did not know. I did know, at that moment on the pier, that it was not up to me. I could not keep Michael alive. I was not in charge of his life and how he had chosen to live it. I was not in charge of his death, anymore than I was in charge of the wind and the waves. And Michael's healing was all about learning to love, especially learning to love his parents all over again, and that lovingness had nothing to do with how long he lived.

Could I surrender the weight of all my personal responsibility for Michael's life, for Michael's happiness, for Michael's healing, from off my own shoulders onto God's shoulders? Could I really trust God to take care of Michael, however that taking care of looked to me, however the future flowed forth? *Surrender* is not a word or a process that comes easily to me. Yet now I had no choice except to trust. My human efforts made as little difference as trying to stem the tides. And so I let Michael go. I gave him over, out of my human hands and heart.

I turned, inevitably, to the other side of the marina. There was the stillness, the peacefulness, the safety. There was the other side of the ocean. There were the "still waters" that would "restore my soul." I don't know how many times I repeated the Twenty-third Psalm. But repeat it I did, over and over, a litany of trust, a litany of surrender.

And then I went home and called Michael and told him how much I loved him. I kept on telling him that, afterwards, in every way I knew how. And I left the rest up to God.

The crises we meet are always about life and how we choose to live it. The crises we meet are about fearing forward into the light. The crises we meet are ultimately about love. How we meet it, how we give it, how we receive it, how we behold it in every human being we have contact with. I believe implicitly in the introduction of *A Course in Miracles* wherein it states that our whole purpose in this life is to remove the blocks to love's awareness.

It says in part: "The Course does not aim at teaching the meaning of love, for that is beyond what can be taught. It does aim, however, at removing the blocks to the awareness of love's presence, which is your natural inheritance. The opposite of love is fear, but what is all-encompassing can have no opposite."

The threat of death is a great teacher for all of us. It is an opportunity not only to plumb the depths of our own human experience but also to dare the heights of our own capacity to love, to find out what we truly believe about ourselves and to take that daring, trusting leap into magnificence of heart.

I doubt that there is anyone reading these pages who hasn't experienced death in one form or another. Death of a parent, a friend, a spouse; death of a marriage, a relationship, a dream. We all face death in one way or another, some on a daily basis, some only once or twice in a lifetime.

I remember Louie Nassaney's sister, Adria. (Louie is a young man, now the picture of glowing health, who was diagnosed with AIDS way back in 1982 and now has no visible evidence of AIDS). Adria came to Louise Hay's Thursday night group just eight days after her eight-year-old son had died of a brain tumor. Her brother had lived through AIDS, as had his whole family, and now she had lost her son, instead of her brother, to death. Her courage that night was remarkable, spontaneous, unfeigned. For she was there that night to help *us*! She was there to give of herself movingly and joyfully in a testimony of her beliefs about one's capacity to live in the midst of death. I remember a song she began to sing in a quavering voice, until we all, hesitantly at first, then with resonance and conviction, joined in. It was a song about doors opening and closing in one's life, and that we are, in the midst of the doors closing and the doors opening, safe, because all of life is change.

I remembered the long, lyrical passage I had written in a previous book, honoring and celebrating the seasons of the magnificent, one-hundred-year-old silver leaf maple tree that I could see from the window of my study, in a home I had lived in and loved for so many years, in a life I had lived that was no longer a reality for me, in a home and a life I had lost, a love I had lost. I remembered the mourning I had gone through, the deaths I had experienced within myself.

There is a new tree I can see from my apartment window, here in Santa Monica. It is a sturdy California tree, which, in this season of winter, is bare and stark and devoid of beauty. But it will bloom again. A new tree. A new place for me. A new life.

"I'm not afraid of death," said Michael.

"My brush with death has taught me how to love," said one AIDS person. "It has opened my eyes to the incredible beauty of life."

"My son's death has not been in vain," said one mother to me. "We were able to love one another before he died."

"There is no death. There are only new beginnings," said another.

As I sat in that church pew that Thanksgiving day I knew what I wanted to say. When the opportunity came to express my feelings in a discussion period, I said that I knew what Michael's life, and my part in his life, were all about. "We are taking the stones of tragic experience and turning those stones into the bread of life, into nourishment and sustenance for ourselves and others."

Later Michael called me. He had gone through three days in which his doctor and everyone around him believed he did, indeed, have pneumocystis. A bed had been prepared for him in the hospital. All the hospital had to do was to run a series of X rays to determine the extent of the pneumocystis. The first set of X rays they ran was inconclusive. The second set of X rays they ran didn't come out. As Michael sat in the waiting room he told me that he prayed not to disappoint the members of his group that depended on him. He prayed to be well and healthy so that he could continue to do the counseling work for others that was his life's plan.

"I prayed to live so that I could continue to give," he told me.

The nurse came into the waiting room where Michael sat crying. He thought she had come to show him to his hospital bed. Instead, she had come to tell him that the third set of X rays showed absolutely no signs of pneumocystis. The doctor couldn't believe it. But Michael could. He said that he cried then like he had never cried before.

"I knew then," he told me, "that I need never fear death, that I would be given the time to do the work that I am here for."

I shared with him my feeling on the stones-into-bread insight. "Each of us is doing just that as we go through the AIDS experience with our loved ones. Whatever the outcome, however the doors close, so do they open as well, and open us to new life, new beginnings in the name of love."

Child of God, you were created
to create the good, the beautiful,
and the holy. Do not forget this.
—A COURSE IN MIRACLES

EPILOGUE

When a child dies before his parents, no matter what his age, it violates the order of the universe. My son Michael died on July 14, 1986.

He was surrounded by his loving family: by his ex-stepmother Nancy, by me, and at various times during the last months of his life, by his brothers Bill, John, and Robert, by his grandmother from Texas, and by his father. In addition, Steve, his friend and therapist, was there for him, as well as John, his roommate of several years. Friends called daily. Michael was also receiving devoted care from AIDS/Hospice workers, from Shanti counselors, and from Dr. Ainsworth; yet although he was surrounded with the unconditional love and support he had asked for, still, Michael died.

He died at Nancy's house, a half block from his own apartment, as he had asked us earlier, choosing to die at home rather than to be kept alive in the impersonality of the hospital. He made a conscious choice during that last month, to let his deteriorating body go, and to let himself go to God. It was an agonizing time for all of us. And we will never be the same again.

For Michael did not "go gently into that good night." To the very end, the human side of Michael fought for control, for mastery, for breath, for life—*life*—while the spiritual side of Michael, who had made his peace weeks before with death, wanted—begged even—to leave the wasted body on the bed and escape gratefully into "that safe and peaceful place where Gee-Gee and Zacky are waiting for me." (Gee-Gee was Michael's great-grandmother and Zacky was Michael's nephew, who had died two years previously.)

How ironic that in the last weeks of Michael's life, we who had prayed so earnestly for Michael to live—"Michael, dear Michael, child of my heart. Don't die!"—now prayed through our tears for his swift release. Again and again the words rose from my heart unspoken. "Michael, dear Michael, child of my heart. Let go! I release you to God, dear child."

For he was a child in those last few weeks. At times he was cross, fretful, angry, demanding, imperious. At times he was an eighty-pound baby, frightened, crying out for his two "mothers." At times he was a childlike spirit coming out of a comatose state to thank us all so politely for taking care of him.

Writing these words, I am reminded daily of that difficult time, when all I believed in about life, about death, about love, was put to the test. And if one sentence that I write can help another mother, another father, another brother or sister or grandmother, another lover or friend or health worker to understand the process of healing—yes, *healing*—in the midst of the process called dying, then Michael's death will not have been in vain. I believe that just as there are alternatives to healing, like the ones Michael explored so diligently, and which resulted in a much longer life span for him than previously predicted, so there are alternatives available in the dying process itself. What we learned in those last few weeks of Michael's life can point the way for another family going through a similar situation.

For this is still a book of hope. This is, indeed, a book of love. And so I close my eyes and recreate the last weeks of Michael's life, not in despair, but in a spirit of hope; go back to that time when everything within me cried out for help in meeting the greatest crisis any mother can face, the death of her child.

There are montages that flicker before my eyes every time I close them, pictures that stand out with a clarity and intensity that match those last weeks the family went through.

John, his brother from Texas, sleeping on the floor night after night, awake in an instant to lead Michael to the bathroom while he was still semi-ambulatory. John and I bathing Michael and Michael's unselfconscious, childlike trust as he let the strong arms of his brother support him and help him with this most private of tasks.

I remember Bill, strong, reliable, tender-hearted Bill, Michael's oldest brother, faithfully transporting family members back and forth to be with Michael, and running errands for Michael for months. He and his family used to take Michael to Golden Gate Park to lie in the sun. They were there for him for months as loving helpers. And I remember Bill near the end, consumed by grief for both his son, Zacky, remourning him, and for Michael. At one point Bill was unable to go up the stairs to Nancy's apartment to tend to his brother; and yet still, still, he was doing all he could. And I remember Bill holding me when Michael died.

I remember Nancy reaching out to me, standing shoulder to shoulder with me, holding hands at Michael's bedside at one point when he had been comatose for fifteen hours and I, sleeping in a chaise lounge in his room, counted the pauses between breaths and willed him onward, to where it would not hurt to breathe. We looked down at his body, struggling to hold on to life. "Michael, dear Michael, child of our hearts. Let go!"

I remember Robert, my youngest son, calling daily,

telling Michael again and again as we held the phone to his ear, "I love you, Spike."

And I remember Michael's grandmother, walking into his room with a smile, dressed in a pastel dress, just off the plane from Texas, with all her love shining through her dear face, and Michael saying to her, "Oh Grandmother, you're finally here. Now I know I am safe."

And I remember Nancy and I, with the help of the Shanti counselor, Karen, resolving old differences and falling into each other's arms saying, "I love you!"

The Shanti counselors and the AIDS/Hospice attendants who came the last few days of Michael's life cared both for Michael and for Nancy and me. They helped immeasurably, and their devotion and unselfish regard for all of us brings tears to my eyes even now. For every family caring for their loved one at home, instead of in the hospital, I would beg you to contact both Shanti and Hospice. They served unstintingly, with love and practicality.

For there were times we did not think we could get through this last awesome task of caring for Michael at home. There were numbing fatigue, occasional outbursts of anger, grief so deep it could not be, and yet somehow *was*, borne, flashes of sheer terror. "Am I strong enough, God, to be here for Michael? Am I strong enough to go through this valley, this shadowed place, with my heart wide open, with my arms wide open?" Bathing Michael, lifting Michael, turning Michael, talking with Michael, listening to Michael, soothing Michael, medicating Michael. "Little bird, open your mouth," and his mouth would obey while the precious drops of morphine dropped in one by one, and then he would go off in a space so far from us that we were surprised each time he came back.

"He's apartment-hunting," explained Frank, another Shanti counselor. "He goes out of his body and looks around and decides where he wants to be. But evidently," and he laughed, "he keeps coming back to Nancy's house because it's the most beautiful, comfortable place he can imagine."

"Let me sing to him while I'm taking care of him," said Sandy, one of the AIDS/Hospice attendants keeping the night vigil. "That will ease him so he won't be afraid." I looked into the room again and again that night, only to see this beautiful black woman kneeling by Michael's bed, holding his hand, while he slept. Her soft lullaby words went on and on, while the candles guttered into dawn.

Within those nights there was time for me, and, I trust, everyone of us, to revise our own feelings about death—time to go through each separate fear and anger and grief about Michael's dying. For although the dying process itself is a hard place inside you that seems to go on and on unbearably, unmercifully, an ordeal that seems never to end, while watching your child die is the hardest task any of us will ever have to face; still, past the struggle there is death, merciful death, not to be dreaded, but to be welcomed. I said to myself again and again during those weeks, "Death is nothing to fear. Death is a kind friend."

The human spirit is resilient. The human spirit *is* love. Each of us had hourly opportunities to question and to experience the intensity of our feelings and the validity of our beliefs. We were challenged in each moment to *be* the love, the absolute, no-holds-barred, unconditional love that Michael had asked for. We were forced again and again to stretch ourselves to the limit of endurance, to the limit of love as we knew it.

And there were times when Michael himself was luminous. I remember an earlier visit, in June, when he sat by the fire in Nancy's living room, with a shawl around him, and we laughed and talked and were happy together. For it was a joy to be in his presence and I want always to remember those moments, when Michael was more spirit than flesh, and yet, and yet, more alive, more *here*, more in the immediacy of the moment, than I had ever seen him. We amazed ourselves at those times, at our laughter, at our spontaneous expressions of affection, at our own tenderness and vulnerability and again—peacefulness—as Michael began to let go of his earthly form.

Michael had asked for three things to happen when he discovered he had AIDS.

He asked that everyone in his family be healed. Oh dearest Michael, that has come true! I remember Hedy, the head AIDS/Hospice nurse, leaning over him, whispering to him as she tried to find out what was holding Michael back from release during the last days of his life; what was holding him in this pattern of shuttling between the worlds of life and death, and understanding instinctively that he felt that he had not said goodbye to everyone. "Ah Michael," she said gently, as he looked into her eyes and tried to make his wishes articulate. "All you have to do is say goodbye in your heart. And that person will know you love and forgive him." An expression of peace passed over Michael's face and he fell asleep.

The second thing that Michael had asked for was to be surrounded by unconditional love. During the last years of his life, everyone he knew cared deeply about him, from his workmates to his friends, to the helpers that attended him, to every member of his family, No one could have experienced more love than Michael did up to the last moments of his life. And that love continues even now.

The third thing that Michael asked for was to be able to do the work that was his to do. When I first began writing this book, Michael was ablaze with enthusiasm. He envisioned himself reaching out to others who had AIDS. He saw himself telling his story, unafraid, risking his self through telling the truth about his illness. More importantly, he wanted to share his deepest self in courage and in love. He talked often about the awakening that AIDS had brought into his life, the 180 degree turn-around that had led him into a deepening relationship with God. He wanted to make a difference in the world.

"AIDS has removed the barriers between me and other people. AIDS is the catalyst that has taught me how to love."

He believed at the time that he *would* live. I believed this too. In fact, there was a time when Michael thought himself to be a failure *because* his physical body was obviously deteriorating, despite all his efforts to heal himself within and without by every means available to him at that time. This trap of spiritual pride, wherein you are "good" if you demonstrate health and "bad, wrong, a failure," if the body does not follow your commands, was a hard lesson for Michael to learn. He went through a time of profound anguish, continually seeking to understand, continually seeking peace at a deeper level, and finally, I trust, letting go of the belief that insisted that healing was limited to the physical body and that "not healing" the physical body meant failure.

"Facts are the enemy of Truth," said Don Quixote. This is a statement that has helped me to understand that Michael's healing *was* accomplished. It is true that the physical body of Michael, after more than two years with the AIDS diagnosis, did, in fact, consume itself. And it is equally true that Michael will live forever—in our hearts, in our minds, in our souls.

I like to think that Michael did, indeed, get his last wish—that of making a difference in the world through telling his story with courage and love.

I remember one of the nights I was sleeping in his room, with the lamp turned down so low that there were only shadows in the room, except for the light that fell upon Michael. Around midnight, dozing in and out of a fretful sleep, the little voice came from the bed. "Mama, Mama."

I roused myself. After I had tended to his physical

needs and kissed him and smoothed his hair back from his childlike, cadaverous face, he gestured for the legal pad and pen we used to write down his medications. It was extremely hard for Michael to speak at this point. The Kaposi's Sarcoma had taken over the roof of his mouth and his throat so that he could not eat, could barely swallow. He spoke slowly, croakily, urgently.

"Write—this—down—Mama.—Write this—down."

I obediently took the pad and pen and waited, poised. Michael often dictated his requests to us, and we laughingly said that he would stay in control through his dictation process until his last breath.

I understood immediately that Michael's mind was wandering and that he thought I was still writing the book about his life. He had often questioned me in the last few weeks about some minor points in the book, chiefly those that dealt with the changes that had taken place within him both physically and emotionally, since the book had first been published in an earlier edition.

"Write—this—down—Mama.—NOW.—Write this down."

He dictated slowly, with long pauses between words.

"I, Michael,—am peaceful—now.—Because—I am not—yelling—at my mother—anymore.— Because—I love—and—appreciate—her—so."

I waited, tears steaming down my face, for more. What did Michael have to say that was so urgent that it could bring him back to coherence, however briefly, with such urgency? What words were there to leave the world to remember him by?

But there was only silence.

I touched Michael's face. He was sleeping peacefully. All trace of tension was gone from his face. I did not know it then, but except for a few disconnected phrases, Michael would not speak coherently again.

Yet in that early morning moment, Michael told me

what I most needed to hear. That he was peaceful. That his struggle was over. And that he loved me. His message was not for the whole world. And yet I share it with you now. "I love you." As he did us all.

I love you too, Michael. And I always will. Sleep, little one.

You are safe. It's only change. Go forward in love.

Bibliography

Books

AIDS Project, Los Angeles. *Living With AIDS: A Self-Care Manual*. California: AIDS PROJECT/Los Angeles, Inc., 1986.

Cousins, Norman. *Anatomy of an Illness: As Perceived by the Patient*. New York: Norton, 1979.

————. *The Healing Heart: Antidotes to Panic and Helplessness*. New York: Norton, 1983.

Foundation for Inner Peace. *A Course in Miracles*. New York: Coleman Graphics, 1975.

Hay, Louise. *You Can Heal Your Life*. California: Hay House, 1986.

Keyes, Ken. *The Hundredth Monkey*. California: Living Love Publications, 1984.

Jampolsky, Gerald G. *Teach Only Love: The Seven Principles of Attitudinal Healing*. New York: Bantam Books, 1983.

Matthews-Simonton, Stephanie, O. Carl Simonton, and James L. Creighton. *Getting Well Again*. New York: Bantam Books, 1980.

Ramsay, Ronald W., M.D., and Rene Noorbergen. *Living With Loss: A Dramatic New Breakthrough in Grief Therapy*. New York: William Morrow & Company, Inc., 1981.

Ray, Sondra. *Celebrations of Breath*. California: Celestial Arts, 1985.

Periodicals and Pamphlets

Bolen, Jean Shinoda, M.D. "William Calderon: Incredible Triumph Over AIDS Brings New Hope." *New Realities*. March/April, 1985.

Brooks, Robert N., M.D., "BEING WELL—BEING GAY— AIDS." Pamphlet. 1985.

Cousins, Norman. "Survival as an Option." *New Realities*. January/February, 1985.

Kessler, David, R.N. "Precautions for Health Care Workers." Pamphlet. 1985.

"Statistics of Health Care Workers." *Journal of the AMA*, Volume 254, #15, October 18, 1985.

Tapes

Hay, Louise. *AIDS: A Positive Approach*. Audio. Hay House. 1985.

————. *Doors Opening: A Positive Approach to AIDS*. Video. Hay House. 1986.

Resources

AIDS/Hospice VNA of San Francisco. 225 30th St., San Francisco, California 94131. Tel: (415) 285-5622.

AIDS Project/Los Angeles, Inc., 7362 Santa Monica Boulevard, Los Angeles, California, 90046. Tel: (213) 876-8951.

Being Well—Being Gay—AIDS. Robert N. Brooks, M.D., 9201 Sunset Boulevard, Suite 718, Los Angeles, California 90069. Tel. (213) 271-4556.

Center for Attitudinal Healing. Gerald Jampolsky, M.D., Tiburon, California.

Expect a Miracle. James C. Baker, 790 California Street, Suite 37, San Francisco, California 94108. Tel. (415) 781-1928.

Love Your Self—Heal Your Body. c/o Hay House, 1242 Berkeley Street, Suite 6, Santa Monica, California 90404 Tel. (213) 828-3666.

Inner Beauty Services. BettyClare Moffatt, 2339 28th Street, Santa Monica, California 90405. Tel. (213) 450-6485.

Love Heals. P.O. Box 480367, Los Angeles, California 90048. Tel. (213) 829-5947.

Parrish, Steve, certified rebirther, 1232 Harvard Street, Suite 12, Santa Monica, California 90404. Tel. (213) 829-5947.

Progressive Nursing Services. David Kessler, R.N., 10680 West Pico Boulevard, Suite 220, Los Angeles, California 90064. Tel. (213) 838-5050.

Shanti Foundation. (213) 273-7591.

Shanti Project. 890 Hayes St., San Francisco, California 94131 (415) 285-5622.

Simonton Cancer Center. (213) 459-4434.

Author's Note: I would like to hear from you. May I invite you to answer these questionnaries? All replies will be confidential. Use additional sheets if necessary. Write as much as you feel comfortable with. Thank you!

BettyClare Moffatt
LOVE HEALS / IBS PRESS
2339 28th Street
Santa Monica, CA 90405

QUESTIONNAIRE I

For Persons Who Have or Had AIDS

1. What were your initial reactions when you were first diagnosed as having AIDS?

2. How did other people react to your AIDS diagnosis (especially your family)?

3. Describe the medical course of your illness and doctor's comments in as much detail as you feel comfortable with.

4. When and how did you decide to live? Describe your emotional insights and thought processes in as much detail as possible.

5. What kinds of alternate therapies did you choose? (Diet, nutrition, homeopathic, chiropractic, support groups, etc.)? Are you continuing these alternate therapies?

6. What advice can you offer to others who contract AIDS and/or the people involved with the AIDS person (relatives, coworkers, etc.)? What would you like to tell the general public, including the media?

7. Why did you choose AIDS? How has this illness served you? What are you going to do for the rest of this life you have chosen to live?

QUESTIONNAIRE II

For Parents, Coworkers, Friends, Support Personnel, etc., of People Who Have AIDS

1. What were your initial reactions upon learning that _____ had AIDS?

2. How did the AIDS person react to you and to others? Describe reactions of family members, friends, doctors, etc. Describe your reactions to their reactions.

3. Describe your emotional insights and thought processes concerning your loved one's AIDS journey. What helped you most? What helped you least?

4. Has this illness changed your attitudes toward life and death? What other attitudes have changed as a result of the AIDS illness? How has this illness served them, you, and others?

5. What advice can you offer to other parents, friends, health professionals, etc., whose loved ones contract AIDS? What advice can you offer to the general public?

6. (Optional) Describe medical procedures and alternative therapies (diet, nutrition, homeopathic, chiropractic, support groups, etc.) that the AIDS person utilized. What kind of help are you now receiving?